6/70

D1191175

IN THE NAME OF MENTAL HEALTH

RONALD LEIFER, M.D.

IN

THE NAME OF

MENTAL HEALTH

The Social Functions of Psychiatry

SCIENCE HOUSE   NEW YORK

To Betty

Contents

IN THE NAME OF MENTAL HEALTH

Preface

━━━━━

Recent developments in psychiatric theory and practice, namely, social and community psychiatry, have led many psychiatrists to modify or abandon the concept of mental illness. In addition, the concept of mental illness has been strongly criticized as inappropriate for understanding psychiatric "patients." Whether psychiatric "patients" are to be viewed as suffering from diseases or as experiencing some other kind of problem is important. If the problems with which psychiatrists deal are not to be viewed as diseases, perhaps psychiatrists should not be viewed as physicians who diagnose, treat, and prevent mental illness.

If psychiatrists are not to be viewed as physicians, then how are they to be viewed? What is the nature and function of psychiatry—of the mental hospital, of psychotherapy, of psychiatric courtroom testimony, of community psychiatry and of other psychiatric activities? The chief purpose of this book is to describe in nonmedical terms the social functions of psychiatry.

This task is complicated by numerous pressures to continue using the medical model in psychiatry—to continue viewing psychiatrists as physicians and their clients as patients who are mentally ill. The image of psychiatry is so deeply permeated with medical rhetoric that to describe psychiatry without using medical terms requires resisting compelling habits of thought and language.

Psychiatrists, as a group, have a substantial investment in

a medical view of psychiatry. The concept of mental illness is not used only because of its intellectual or scientific value. This concept is central to the psychiatrist's identity as a physician. If the concept of mental illness were to be rejected as an inept metaphor for describing certain kinds of human behavior, the psychiatrist would be cast adrift in a sea of obsolete fictions. His aims, methods, and concepts would have to be reinterpreted. Perhaps he would have to forge a new social identity.

Society also has an investment in the medical view of psychiatry. By using the medical model to describe and explain them, certain *social* activities may be performed as medical services. When viewed as social rather than medical, the moral and political character of psychiatric activities would come more clearly into focus for the public to see. The nature of psychiatry might then become a public question. Practices that are accepted when defined as medical might be rejected when defined as social, moral, or political.

Because the medical view of psychiatry has social utility, resistance to a critique of this view is to be expected. This resistance follows the classical patterns of the opposition of established social interests to unsettling ideas. Ideas, including social theories, occur in the context of social life and have social value. Some ideas will suit the interests of one group or another, others will threaten those interests, and still others will be considered irrelevant or trivial. To understand a concept properly, it is necessary to understand its relation to social life. A social description of psychiatric practices will be in competition with a medical description of those practices. An account of the social functions of psychiatry must therefore include an analysis of the social utility of the medical model, its relation to psychiatric practices and to social life in general.

As a social institution, the primary purpose of psychiatry is to provide services—to act in the affairs of men. This purpose provides the guiding thread of psychiatric thought. As a group, psychiatrists belong to a specialized, professional subculture that functions in a particular historical, economic, and political matrix. They have a common training and social identity, and their prestige and livelihood depend upon properly fulfilling professionally defined obligations. Psychiatric thought tends to express, justify, and advance the purposes and programs of organized psychiatry.

Like the members of other social groups, psychiatrists tend to speak, think and act within the limits in which rewards are provided and punishments avoided. The inducements to thought and action, or to their avoidance, are provided by social instruments of power and control which, in effect, bribe and threaten the individual to perform properly. As with other social groups, inquiry that furthers psychiatric group identity, aims, and interests is approved. Inquiry that challenges them may be disapproved or even punished.

While understandable, such a situation is unfortunate. If psychiatry is to function as a science and advance our understanding of man, it must balance its service obligations with vigorous intellectual inquiry and self-criticism. To do this, it is necessary to encourage personal freedom—not only for psychiatric patients, but also for psychiatrists themselves. That inquiry has a personal element must be recognized. Understanding is mediated by personal experiences and ultimately serves personal interests. For some these experiences and interests are intimately bound to professional life. For others they are not. Each man should be free to search for what he seeks and to believe in what he finds.

While writing this book, I have enjoyed discussions with many psychiatric colleagues who have themselves expressed or agreed with ideas presented here. I have also enjoyed discussions with colleagues whose views differ from mine but who nevertheless encouraged my inquiries. I owe my chief intellectual debts to Freud, Dewey, Mannheim, and Wittgenstein, and to my friends and teachers Thomas Szasz, Ernest Becker, Stanley Diamond, and Alfred Louch. I confess to having exploited them thoroughly by borrowing from them ideas that I found congenial to my own intellectual development and temperament. Since each was my teacher, the attentive reader may see the thoughts of these men balanced off against one another. What they may charge to be distortions of their views, I readily admit to be the result of the liberties I have taken with their work.

Most authors owe some personal debt of gratitude to those who have helped him to live the life of a writer. My gratitude is deepest to my wife Betty, who has provided me with a loving atmosphere in which I could attempt to think and live creatively. I am also grateful to the American Council of Learned Societies for expressing confidence in my work with a generous financial grant. I wish to express my appreciation to Seymour Weingarten, my editor at *Science House*, and to Laura Frazee, who ably edited the manuscript. Finally, I wish to thank my friends Roger Yanow and T. Patterson Brown for reading the manuscript, making helpful suggestions, and permitting me to use their reactions to my work as a guide for its style.

PART ONE

A Theoretical Perspective on Psychiatry

CHAPTER ONE

Psychiatry and the Medical Model

. . . a large part of thinking and knowing cannot be correctly understood, as long as its connection with existence or with the social implications of human life are not taken into account.

—KARL MANNHEIM[1]

Psychiatry is usually defined as a medical specialty that diagnoses, treats, and prevents mental illness. This definition is more than a simple description. It suggests that psychiatry should be viewed as a medical activity.

There are a number of reasons for thinking of psychiatry as a medical activity. Psychiatry has close historical connections with medicine. It is an offspring of neurology, that branch of medicine dealing with diseases of the nervous system. Consequently, all psychiatrists are physicians. Psychiatrists are licenced by the state to practice medicine, they function within the framework of organized medicine, and their social identity lies in their medical credentials. As a discipline, psychiatry is taught only in medical schools as are pediatrics, surgery, and radiology.

The setting, the props and the rhetoric of the psychiatric pageant are strongly medical. Psychiatrists often work in clinics, offices and hospitals with other physicians. These psychiatrists may dress in white, carry medical instruments, and perform diagnostic and therapeutic services, particularly in neurology, in which they are required to receive special training to be accredited by the American Board of Psychiatry and Neurology. Some aspects of psychiatric practice are similar to regular medical procedures. Psychiatrists administer drugs, electro-shock, and insulin. Finally, psychiatrists may do research in neurophysiology, neuropharmacology, or other aspects of the bodily process.

The rhetoric of psychiatric theory and practice is also strongly medical. Persons who consult psychiatrists are called "patients." They complain of "symptoms" and suffer from "diseases." The psychiatrist's inquiries are called "examinations" and lead him to "diagnoses." The services he renders are labelled as "treatments." They often take place in "hospitals" and, hopefully, lead to "remissions" and "cures." Such rhetoric seems to support the view of psychiatry as a medical activity.

The medical view of psychiatry has been firmly established as a habit of thinking, cemented by custom, convention, and precedent and buttressed by huge financial commitments. Numerous private and public organizations spend much money, time, and energy to convince the general public that the person with mental illness is sick, as is a person with any other disease and that mental illness is a major health problem that claims as many as one person in ten as its victim and fills every other hospital bed with those who suffer from its effects. The wide acceptance of these claims by both the general public and the medical profession is an important factor in the success of the medical view of psychiatry.

Nevertheless, there are significant differences between the intellectual interests and professional activities of psychiatrists and other physicians. These differences raise questions about viewing psychiatry as a medical activity. To begin, no matter what the intermediate concerns of psychiatrists, the ultimate concern is with human consciousness and behavior. Psychiatric interest in bodily mechanisms is always with an eye to their influence on mind and behavior. The reverse is true in medicine where interest in mind and behavior is for the purpose of understanding and manipulating the body. Every medical specialty except psychiatry has in common an ultimate interest in the structure and function of the human body as a physicochemical machine; these specialties serve their patients by intervening in bodily processes. Psychiatrists, on the other hand, are interested in and intervene in human behavior and social processes.

The theoretical concerns of psychiatrists differ markedly from those of their nonpsychiatric colleagues. Psychiatrists are concerned with a scope of the human drama that is matched perhaps only by the artist and general essayist of the human condition. Psychiatrists are considered to be experts on the panorama of human consciousness, the passions, and the complete cycle of life from birth through maturation, procreation, marriage, work, recreation, and aging to death. They ponder and pontificate on the total range of human activity and expression from language, art, myth, religion, and law to propaganda, war, crime, and the deeds of great and ordinary men. Finally, psychiatrists study and advise us about the troubles of our times—poverty, delinquency, illiteracy, the cold war, the menace of nuclear holocaust—and the future of civilization.

This range of the psychiatrist's intellectual interests is equalled by the range of his social involvements. Psychiatrists converse, counsel, advise, persuade, and analyze persons who have problems not with their bodies, but with the personal and social dimensions of their lives. They attempt to mend broken marriages, rehabilitate criminals, and counsel delinquents. They advise welfare departments, adoption agencies, and poverty programs. They screen, teach, and advise Peace Corps Volunteers, military personnel, and government employees. They help to promote industrial advertising, sales, and personnel efficiency. They attempt to improve the education of the under-achieving student and to affect the morals of the sexually confused collegian. Psychiatrists testify in courtrooms about who is and is not competent to stand trial. to make a will, to enter a contract, or to go to prison. They administer and staff institutions in which psychiatric patients are held against their will. Finally, they have become concerned with alleviating the distresses of social life and with devising and promoting social programs to eliminate poverty, delinquency, illiteracy, unemployment, and boredom.[2]

The view of psychiatry as a medical activity is known as the medical model of psychiatry. The similarities between psychiatry and medicine tend to justify the use of the medical model of psychiatry. The differences between them tend to call into question the credibility and the utility of that model. Whether the similarities between psychiatry and medicine are to be considered more important than their differences, and, hence, whether the medical model is to be employed does not depend solely on scientific considerations. It depends also on social factors.

Conceptual models, such as the medical model of psychiatry serve both scientific and social functions. To the degree that models "fit" (or are metaphorically apt to) the terrain they map, they serve the *scientific function* of helping us to understand our subject matter.[3] To the degree that conceptual models facilitate, avoid interference with, or obstruct the practical tasks of living, they have a *social function*. Hence, the acceptance or rejection of models depends on both scientific and social factors.

THE SCIENTIFIC FUNCTIONS OF THE MEDICAL MODEL OF PSYCHIATRY

The medical model of psychiatry has two related aspects. It is a conceptual scheme for understanding psychiatrists, and it is a model for understanding psychiatric patients.

As a scheme for understanding psychiatrists, the medical

model views them as physicians who function as do other physicians to diagnose, treat and prevent (mental) disease. According to this model, they do this by reducing or eliminating disease-causing stresses or by increasing the patient's capacities to adapt successfully to those stresses.

As a scheme for understanding psychiatric patients, the medical model views human behavior in terms of the biological and medical concepts of homeostasis, health, and disease. According to these concepts, organismic life and functions are maintained within a precariously balanced range of conditions. Potentially hostile agents in the external and internal environment may upset this balance. An individual who is exposed to these agents, which range from physical, chemical, and organic to psychological and sociocultural stresses, may fall victim to them if his resistances fall below a certain level. Disease is thus construed as a disordered state of bodily function, mind, or behavior that is the result of the failure to adapt to stress.

A conceptual model may aid our understanding of a particular subject even when the fit is not exact. For instance, we use the planetary metaphor to explain the revolution of electrons about an atomic nucleus even though evidence suggests electron clouds rather than discrete orbiting entities. Indeed, since scientific models are metaphors that compare unfamiliar events to familiar events, the fit is seldom exact. Often, there are competing models to explain a particular set of phenomena. A model is discarded when omissions, differences, and discrepancies are described between the model and the relevant data and when better fitting alternative models are suggested.

The use of the medical model to conceptualize psychiatric patients and practitioners may be challenged by a critique of the fit of medical and biological concepts to human social behavior. While these concepts may be useful for understanding biological survival and adaptability, their utility for understanding the rules, games, meanings, and values of social action are highly dubious. Alternative models for understanding individual behavior, for instance, the dramatical and the game models, seem better suited to the relevant facts of human experience. Indeed, psychiatrists seem to have accepted alternative models of human behavior for their scientific advantages while simultaneously retaining the medical model for its social advantages.

It should be apparent that the uses of the medical model for explaining the behavior of psychiatric patients and physicians are complementary and interdependent. If human behavioral function and malfunction were viewed in terms of sociological rather than medical and biological models, we would be obliged to abandon the idea that the psychiatrist functions as do other physicians to diagnose, treat, and prevent illness. Conversely, if we could fully explain psychiatric functions in sociological terms, we would be tempted to replace the medical model of the psychiatric patient with a sociological model. It would not be logical to insist that only physicians are qualified to deal with phenomena that we do not regard as illnesses. Nor would it be logical to insist that familiar social operations are, in the special case of the psychiatrist, directed against phenomena that are to be regarded as fundamentally similar to the diseases medical physicians treat by physicochemical means.

THE SOCIAL FUNCTIONS OF THE MEDICAL MODEL OF PSYCHIATRY

Conceptual models (like all other ideas) are not the result of a private romance between the solitary scientist (or thinker) and the object of his study. They are fully social acts that have an historical development, a present context of use, and a future impact. Ideas may serve to justify and perpetuate social interests and functions. Or, ideas may serve to challenge beliefs, to undermine customs, and to generate change. As a result, both subtle and explicit pressures are exerted on model-makers and model-critics to promote or oppose one scheme rather than another. This is particularly true of ideas in the social sciences that emerge directly out of the life and style of a people and, reciprocally, have a direct impact on their self-regard, their social relationships, and their development.

The relationship between ideas and social life is reciprocal. Ideas have an impact on social practices, but social practices also influence the selection and perception of facts and the language used to explain them. Models are conceptual lenses that prepare and inform our perception and expression. In turn, the popularity and success of conceptual models is influenced by social practices and conventions. To understand why a particular idea is embraced or rejected requires that one understand its historical development, the social context in which it is proposed or used, and its impact on social life.

The present use of the medical model of psychiatry cannot be attributed solely to the contemporary psychiatrist's conviction of its logical and empirical correctness. Karl Mannheim held that it is incorrect to say that the single scientist thinks, perceives, and denotes. It is more correct to say that he furthers the thinking, perceiving, and denoting of other men before him.[4] The medical model is the conceptual keystone of modern psychiatry, and psychiatry is an important social institution with a long history, an intricate social context, and complex social functions. The careers of the medical model and of psychiatry as a social institution are intimately intertwined and interdependent. Competing models of human behavioral function and malfunction not only must withstand the falsifying thrusts of experiment and experience but also must prevail against the momentum of habit, custom, and proven social utility. To understand the utility of the medical model in psychiatry we must inquire not only into the logical and empirical justifications for it, but also into the social, economic, and political influences on its development and use. Our analysis of the medical model is thus not merely a task in epistemology and scientific method but also exercise in the sociology of knowledge.[5]

As the keystone of the medical model of psychiatry, the concept of mental illness should help us to understand and organize the facts about an individual's behavior. Although this concept is alleged to be scientific, it is not used by the behavioral scientist in the value neutral (social influence free) atmosphere of his laboratory. The label "mental illness" is not assigned to individuals on the basis of random selection and "objective" study. It is used by the psychiatric practitioner in the complex social circumstances of his practice and must be understood in this context.

It is impossible to understand the nature and function of the medical model until we understand the nature and function of psychiatry as a social institution. This is because psychiatry is the instrument by means of which the medical model is defined and used. This is an affirmation of the principle of Operationism, which holds that the position and interventions of the scientist cannot be divorced from his ideas about the data under study. In physics, the concepts of space and time cannot be construed separately from the corresponding operations by which they are assessed.[6] If the concept-maker functions in a social setting, as the psychiatrist does, then his concepts must be understood in the context of his social situation and his social operations.[7]

This means that the social functions of psychiatry must be conceptualized in other than medical terms. They must be described in the ordinary language of social discourse or in the somewhat more specialized language of social science. For if we attempt to scrutinize psychiatric practices only through the lenses of the medical model we shall fail to see what is filtered out by this model and we shall perceive only that which is congenial to it. We must be aware that, as metaphors, models may help us to see more clearly that which is congenial to their form. They may, however, also disguise or divert from our attention elements of a situation that they do not assimilate.

We must therefore be alert to the possibility that conceptual models serve as disguises. They may obscure important facts, blur inconsistencies, simplify complexities, and prejudice perspectives. Indeed, one of the main principles of the sociology of knowledge is that conceptual models may serve as a ". . . more or less conscious disguise of the real nature of a situation, the true recognition of which would not be in accord with [certain social] interests."[8] (Brackets added.)

A nonmedical description of psychiatry will reveal that medicine and psychiatry differ in every important respect except the rhetoric used to describe them. Medicine is oriented toward nature and the body; psychiatry is oriented toward society and the person. Medical physicians attempt to relieve the suffering and disability of the flesh. Psychiatrists attempt to relieve "spiritual" suffering and to remedy the disabilities of social performance. To the extent that these important differences are disguised by the medical model, it is a strained metaphor that interferes with our full understanding of the role of psychiatry in modern life.

A nonmedical description of psychiatry will further reveal that it consists of social operations that might be viewed as in conflict with our laws and social values. It will reveal psychiatry to be a social practice that consists not of the diagnosis and healing of illness, but of social control, socialization, moral guidance, education, personal consolation, personnel management, and social reconstruction.

The medical model of psychiatry remains in use because it is socially useful to disguise the social functions of psychiatry. The medical model induces us to accept the claim that the psychiatrist functions as a physician, and it induces us to prejudge his activities with the enthusiastic approval that we give to the practice of medicine. It serves our need for an official explanation of psychiatric practices, which, for complex reasons, it is against our interests to understand or to admit publicly. It also serves our need for an official explanation of certain kinds of individual behavior, which, also for complex reasons, it is against our interests to understand or to admit.

In this sense, the medical model of psychiatry is an ideology that disguises the social, legal, and moral relevance of psychiatric operations because their recognition would not be in accord with social interests. This does not mean that psychiatrists conspire to perform socially unacceptable practices. It means that as a society we are playing a trick on our collective selves so that we may have the advantages of certain psychiatric activities without suffering the disadvantages of describing and judging those activities in political, legal, and moral terms.

A full understanding of the medical model, and the reasons for its continued use, is thus inseparable from a full understanding of the social functions of psychiatry. To understand psychiatric operations it is necessary to examine them in their full historical, social, economic and legal dimensions. To do this it is necessary to examine in detail the four principle areas of psychiatric practice: mental hospitalization, psychotherapy, legal psychiatry, and community psychiatry. This treatment of psychiatric practices is not exhaustive.[9] However, those who comprehend these four principle social functions of psychiatry and the utility of the medical model in each will have no difficulty in understanding and evaluating other psychiatric practices.

CHAPTER TWO

The Medical Model as Idea and Ideology

Pure intellection is not a fact in nature; it is a logical fiction which will not really serve even the purpose of technical logic. In reality our knowing is driven and guided at every step by our subjective interests and preferences, our desires, our needs and our ends. These form the motive powers also of our intellectual life.

Reality, therefore, and the knowledge thereof, essentially presuppose a definitely directed effort to know. And, like other efforts, this effort is purposive; it is necessarily inspired by the conception of some good ("end") at which it aims. Neither the question of *Fact*, therefore, nor the question of *Knowledge* can be raised without raising also the question of *Value*.

—F. C. S. Schiller[1]

The view of psychiatry as a medical activity is often defended with the argument that psychiatry and medicine are fundamentally similar and should therefore be conceptualized with the medical model. The proponents of the medical model argue that medical and psychiatric patients are similar because both are victims of disease and that psychiatric and medical physicians are similar because both perform similar diagnostic and therapeutic functions. Or, they argue that the concepts of disease and treatment should be expanded beyond the boundaries of physical medicine to include all of man's coping with evil.

Logical arguments alone seldom influence people or history. People are moved by their interests, in the defense of which they seldom have difficulty formulating logical arguments. Each argument for the fundamental similiarity of psychiatry and medicine may be countered with an argument for their fundamental difference. The relationship between psychiatry and medicine is historical and social rather than logical and scientific.

Nevertheless, it is important to consider these arguments for and against the use of the medical model in psychiatry. They are presented together seldom enough to warrant the effort. More important, it is necessary to give them their due and be done with them so we can examine the deeper ties that bind psychiatry to medicine.

PSYCHIATRY IS FUNDAMENTALLY MORE LIKE MEDICINE THAN DIFFERENT FROM IT

Medical and Psychiatric Patients Are Similar
Because Both Are Victims of Disease

The most important argument for the use of the medical model in psychiatry is the claim that medical and psychiatric patients[2] are similar because both are victims of disease. The form of this claim must alert us to the possibility that seeming similarities between medical and psychiatric situations are actually similarities in the language used to describe them. The claim that both medical and psychiatric patients are diseased itself employs the medical model and thus cannot be used as an argument for its applicability without begging the issue. It is an *example* of how the medical model might be used in psychiatry. The claim that psychiatric patients are mentally ill is the result of the use of the medical model in psychiatry and not an argument in support of that use.

The same is true for the use of other key terms or concepts of the medical model. One cannot justify the use of the medical model by arguing, for instance, that both medical and psychiatric patients suffer from pathology, symptoms, lesions, syndromes, relapses, or undergo cures. Each of these terms prejudices us to look at the data through the lenses of the medical model rather than to argue for the fit of that model to psychiatric situations.

Underlying the claim that medical and psychiatric patients are similar because both are victims of disease is the claim that they are similar because both experience, or are likely to develop, some form of suffering or disability from which they (or others in their behalf) seek relief. This argument assumes the defining quality of disease to be that it causes suffering and disability.

This claim requires close examination. Human suffering is ubiquitous and has various causes and forms. A man may suffer because he has a broken leg or because he has cancer. Some psychiatric patients may suffer because they have actual diseases of the brain, such as syphilis or arteriosclerosis.[3] However, all suffering does not stem from bodily disorder.[4] People may suffer because they have psychological conflicts, because they are poor, because they are persecuted, because they are unfulfilled, and so on. Most psychiatric patients are drawn from people who suffer from these causes while medical patients are drawn from people who suffer from disorders of their bodies.

The use of the generic term "suffering" in all of these cases does not serve a descriptive purpose. It does not describe the physical state of the sufferer, the quality or cause of his suffering, nor the social circumstances in which it occurs. The claim that medical and psychiatric patients are similar because both suffer serves to classify these two groups of people together within the domain of medicine and to separate them from other sufferers. It does not explain why sufferers should be differentially classified in this manner. Far from being an argument in favor of the similarity between medical and psychiatric patients, this claim is definitional and jurisdictional. It *defines* certain sufferers as ill and *assigns* to medicine the jurisdiction for their relief.

The same considerations apply to disability. A person may be disabled by a broken leg, by heart failure, or by blindness. He may also be disabled by ignorance, poverty, laziness, rebelliousness, or by powerful groups that oppress him. The claim that medical and psychiatric patients are similar because they are disabled and therefore ought to be conceptualized with the same model, serves simply to classify certain kinds of disability together, without either explaining or justifying that classification.

Some persons, particularly a growing group of community psychiatrists, claim that *all* forms of human suffering and disability should be viewed as medical and conceptualized according to the medical model. Those who make this claim, however, do not explain why all suffering and disability ought to be conceptualized in medical terms rather than distinguished according to basic differences and conceptualized with a variety of models. Others, particularly the comprehensive theorists, tend to emphasize the similarities between behavior and bodily function rather than to emphasize their differences. These theorists tend to classify together bodily events and behavior, or medical and mental illness, without specifying why they should be classified together rather than separately.

These theorists often admit that medical and psychiatric patients have difficulties with two different aspects of life—physiological functioning and social behavior. However, these theorists then classify these aspects together within the single category of "the biology of life" or "organismic functioning." All organismic functioning is then conceptualized according to the biological model of the homeostatic equilibrium of systems. Social and physical suffering and disability are considered to be failures of homeostasis—as symptons of disease that are caused by harmful internal or external agents.

To fashion an inclusive model of human life, such comprehensive theorists must, unfortunately, systematically ignore critical differences between psychosocial and biophysical phenomena, namely that each is investigated by a different method and described in a different language.[5] The comprehensive theorists must ignore especially that (the language of) psychosocial behavior has ethical and political dimensions while (the language of) physical events do not. A feature of comprehensive theories in the life sciences therefore, is that they are cryptoethical: They tend to disguise the ethical dimensions of human social life in the value-free lexicon of physics and animal biology.

A scientific model, however, cannot enlighten our understanding by obscuring facts—by obscuring important differences among classes of phenomena. When the differences among classes of phenomena are important to understanding them we require either divergent conceptual models or a single model that permits the assimilation and conceptual organization of those differences. The coclassification of all forms of suffering and disability and of behavioral acts and bodily events does obscure important differences between these classes of phenomena and between medical and psychiatric patients.

Classification does not depend solely on the qualities of the objects or events classified. Similarities and differences exist between any two objects or events in the universe. Classification is a human activity that depends, also, on the purposes of the classifier.[6] To understand why psychiatrists coclassify different forms of suffering and disability, social and physical events, and ethical and nonethical activity, we must understand the purposes of the classifiers.

The standard arguments for the use of the medical model in psychiatry either employ that model subtly or explicitly as the sole argument for its use, or they emphasize similarities between medical and psychiatric patients without offering reasons for that emphasis. When the application of the medical model is thought to carry with it the justification for psychiatric jurisdiction, the global application of the medical model cannot be viewed merely as a scientific exercise that serves to organize or explain data. It must be considered, also, a rhetorical device for classifying certain events as medical in nature to justify psychiatric interventions in them.

The concept of disease is the keystone of the medical model. For the generic term "disease" to be applicable to both medicine and psychiatry there must be similarities between medical and mental illness. Any criticism of the medical model in psychiatry must therefore begin with an elucidation of the differences between medical and mental illness.[7] The paradigmatic argument against the use of the medical model in psychiatry is contained in Thomas Szasz's book *The Myth of Mental Illness*.[8] Let us summarize the main points of his argument.

The main component of Szasz's argument is that the conceptual problems surrounding the medical model and the concept of mental illness are linguistic. That is to say, they derive from confusions and ambiguities in the use of language. The first point to be understood is that the term "disease" is neither a mental nor a bodily state. It is a word, the use of which is governed by linguistic and social conventions.[9] As is true of other words, the term "disease" may be employed for different purposes. It may be used for scientific (or cognitive) purposes to convey information. Or it may be used for social purposes to induce feelings and images or to promote action.[10] Words may be used for combinations of purposes or for different purposes at different times under different conditions. Also, the use of words may change. Thus, a man who is labelled a Jew may change his name and relabel himself a non-Jew. Similarly, phenomena labelled as "sin," "crime," or "possession" may be relabelled as "mental illness."[11]

In medicine, the term "disease" serves to convey a particular type of information. What does it tell us? *In every case in which this term is used in medicine* (but not in psychiatry) *it refers to an undesired bodily state.* While physicians may distinquish between lung disease, kidney disease, eye disease, and so on, the common element in all of these situations is some change in bodily structure and function. The generally accepted undesirability of this change is the basis for the ascription of "disease." Thus, the paradigmatic cognitive use of the term "disease" is to denote an undesirable bodily state.

A second cognitive use of the term "disease" is to refer to a social role, namely the role of the ill person.[12] This role constitutes a socially defined *behavior* pattern, which involves certain social exemptions as well as certain social expectations. When it is said that medicine deals with diseased persons, it is sometimes meant that medicine deals with persons whose bodily states have been diagnosed as diseased; at other times it is meant that medicine deals with persons to whom the role of illness has been ascribed; and sometimes it is meant that medicine deals with persons who fall into both of these categories.

The term "disease" is used socially (or promotively, when it permits (or sometimes obligates) a person to assume the social role of the ill person. It is important to note that this use of the word "disease" makes a social pair of the physician and the patient for the physician is the appropriate social alter of the patient. To use the medical model in psychiatry implies that a certain patterned social relationship is formed between persons labelled as "mentally ill" and persons who are called "doctors." In this relationship, the patient is entitled to be treated with kindness and care, to be held not accountable for his disability and to be excused from certain social responsibilities. It also obligates him to seek the aid of a physician and to follow his recommendations.[13] The physician, on the other hand, is charged with the responsibility of providing medical treatment and to avoid doing harm to his patient. The relationship also gives the physician charismatic and (especially in psychiatry) social power over his patient.

The various uses of the term "disease" are independent.

A person might exhibit a diseased body without assuming the social role of illness if, for instance, he were a Christian Scientist or a Stoic. Conversely, a person might be physically healthy but still assume the social role of illness if, for instance, he were a malingerer or a hypochondriac.

Social as well as medical factors determine the uses of the word "disease." In the sense in which the term refers to an undesirable bodily state (as opposed to a social role), it is ascribed to a person by a physician when a physical examination reveals the presence of certain undesirable bodily conditions. In the sense in which the term refers to a social role, its use depends on the decisions and the relative social power of the patient and the physician. Most commonly, the patient with a physical disease will agree to assume the social role of the ill person. However, the patient and the physician may not agree on the patient's role. For instance, the patient without physical disease may wish to assume the sick role and the physician may decline to ascribe it to him. In such cases, the label of malingerer is likely to be assigned to the rejected patient.[14] Or, the physician may wish to define the patient as sick and the patient may refuse. In this situation, the physician and the patient do not necessarily have equal power. The patient may have his way (if his physical condition permits) and refuse to assume the sick role, or the physician may define that person as ill and force him into the social role of patienthood against his will.

The successful promotive use of the label "disease" thus depends on the relative social power of the physician (or the persons or group for whom he is acting as agent) and the patient. It is more difficult to assign an individual the role of illness if he is wealthy, socially prominent, or influential.[15] It is easier if he is a member of the military service, if he is a prisoner, or if he is poor.[16]

There are two striking differences between the uses of the term "disease" in medicine and psychiatry. First, in medicine, the term refers to an undesirable bodily state. In psychiatry it does not, since psychiatric patients have personal and social troubles rather than troubles with their bodies. Thus, the scientific (cognitive, descriptive) use of the term "disease" in psychiatry is always to refer to social behavior.

Second, the medically ill person usually may refuse to accept the social role of illness, if he is physically capable of doing so, without having the competence of his choice impuned and the role thrust upon him against his will. In psychiatry, on the other hand, it is possible for the term "disease" to be ascribed to a person *in order* to introduce him into the social role of illness or *in order* to justify the social action others take against him. Thus, the promotive use of the term "disease" in psychiatry may "promote" involuntary hospitalization, the loss of a job, the refusal of admission to or suspension from school, the refusal of the right to stand trial for a crime of which one has been accused, and so on.

Let us now consider how the term "mental" is used in connection with the word "disease." To employ the term "mental" at all in a scientific context introduces complex logical problems that have an important bearing on the use of the medical model in psychiatry. The term "mental" in psychiatric usage, most often refers to other persons' minds.[17] However, other persons' minds are not objects to be observed by anyone. Other persons' minds are private experiences of their own, about which we can have knowledge only by drawing conclusions from their behavior, including their verbal behavior.[18] This implies that psychiatrists draw conclusions about the mental state (or mental illness) of individuals on the basis of the behavior of those indviduals. Strictly speaking, therefore, when the term "mental" is used in psychiatric discussions, it refers to behavior.

One implication of this is that in medicine the term "disease" refers to phenomena that are not regulated by social custom, morality, and law, namely bodily structure and function. In psychiatry, however, the term "disease" refers to behavior, which *is* subject to the regulation of custom, morality, and law. *This means not only that psychiatric practices may* conflict with law and morality, but also that they may be employed by legal and moral interests as a method of controlling and influencing human behavior. When a physician treats pneumonia he may achieve a moral goal—the preservation of life and bodily function—but he does not enforce moral codes. When the psychiatrist treats a dangerous "schizophrenic" he also may achieve a moral goal—the protection of the welfare and safety of his community—but he also enforces moral and legal codes that prohibit violent acts.

When the word "disease" is used in medicine to refer to undesirable alterations of bodily structure and function, the companion terms indicate the part of the body affected. Kidney disease refers to the kidney, heart disease to the heart, and so on. To what part of the body does the word "mental" refer when it is used in connection with the word "illness?" It would be absurd to answer: "The term 'mental illness' indicates that the part of the body that is diseased is the mind (or behavior)." The mind is not a part of the body, nor is behavior. (The term "mental illness," as it is used here, does not refer to brain disease.) Thus, the medical model in psychiatry is either absurd, because it regards the mind as a part of the body, or the medical model has a very different significance in psychiatry than it does in medicine, since it does not refer to the body at all.

If we grant that in its paradigmatic cognitive use in medicine the term "disease" refers to the body, to modify it with the word "mental" is at worst a mixture of logical levels called a category error, and at best it is a radical redefinition of the word "disease." A category error is an error in the use of language that, in turn, produces errors in thinking. The difference between a word at the logical level of "mind" (or "behavior") and a word at the logical level of the "body" (or "object") may be illustrated with an example from Gilbert Ryle's book The Concept of Mind, which has been instrumental in clarifying a widely accepted modern philosophical position on the mind-body problem.

Ryle describes a child who witnessed a parade of an army

division. After having seen the battalions, batteries, and squadrons, the child asked when the division would appear. He did not appreciate the fact that "soldiers" and "division'" are two different kinds of words, which here have the same meaning. He assumed therefore, that he could see a parade of soldiers followed by the parade of a division. He saw both the parade of soldiers and the parade of a division, but he did not see two events. The soldiers constituted the division.[19]

To assume that the mind is another part of the body that can become diseased, as can the heart and kidneys, is similar to assuming that a division is an additional group of soldiers. One may, and indeed must, understand both the body and the mind as one may understand the character of individual soldiers as well as of divisions. One cannot, however, treat divisions as if they were extra soldiers, nor minds as if they were parts of bodies. Whatever the mind may be, it is not a thing like muscles, bones, and blood.

If the term "disease" is to retain its medical meaning to refer to alterations of the body, then "mental" cannot intelligibly modify it. For the phrase "mental disease" would then be roughly equivalent to "nonphysical alterations of the body." To avoid this difficulty, when the term "illness" is used in psychiatry it should be recognized that it assumes a meaning different from that in medicine: It assumes the meaning of undesirable alterations of behavior. The adjective "mental" serves to indicate that this meaning is in force, that an individual's behavior rather than his body is being referred to. The medical model in psychiatry thus has a metaphorical use: the presentation of facts about human behavior in the idiom of facts pertaining to the human body. As such, the medical model distracts us from an important difference between medicine and psychiatry, namely that the former deals with undesirable states of the body and the latter deals with undesirable patterns of behavior.

This argument for the use of the medical model in psychiatry suffers from three defects. First, it is circular because it uses the medical model in the argument for its use by claiming that psychiatric patients should be classified with medical patients because both suffer from disease. Second, the argument is incomplete because it does not explain why certain kinds of suffering and disability should be classified together rather than separately. Third, it is obscurantist because it obscures the differences between different kinds of suffering and disability, between physical and behavioral (social) events, between the body and behavior, and between the practice of medicine and the practice of psychiatry.

The principle advantages of this argument are therefore neither scientific nor intellectual. They are social. They prejudice the lay public to see psychiatric practices as more like medical treatment than like social control, socialization, education, and religious consolation. It bids them to presume that the psychiatrist, like other physicians, always serves the individual in his pursuit of life, health, and happiness.

Medical and Psychiatric Patients Are Similar Because the Causes of Their Diseases Are Similar

A number of the proponents of the use of the medical model in psychiatry claim that most, or all, mental illnesses will eventually be demonstrated to spring from organic malfunctions of the brain. They maintain that these mental illnesses will be discovered to be varieties of organic brain disease and, thus, to belong to the science and practice of medicine to study and alter. This argument for the use of the medical model in psychiatry is therefore based on the prospect of future proof.

It is true, of course, that as the techniques of neurophysiological research are refined new organic brain diseases are likely to be discovered. It is conceivable, or even likely, that some cases presently diagnosed as schizophrenia will fall into this category (". . . although the search for a biochemical etiology of schizophrenia has been the most notoriously and embarrassingly unproductive research in medicine").[20] It is already known that the brain, like any other organ, may become diseased and that diseases of the brain may adversely influence behavior. The discovery that certain behavior patterns are associated with lesions of the brain would not demonstrate that all mental illnesses have an organic etiology. It would simply demonstrate that we do not know all there is to know about the human body, particularly about diseases of the brain. Moreover, persons with brain disease are medically ill, since they are similar to other medical patients in that alteration of tissue structure and function is associated with their suffering and disability. Therefore, the discovery of new brain diseases will constitute the discovery of new medical illnesses and not the proof that mental illness has an organic etiology.

The argument for the use of the medical model in psychiatry, however, is sometimes based on a stronger claim than that *some* mental illnesses *may be* discovered to be associated with medical illnesses. It is based on the claim that eventually *all* mental events will be reducible to physiological correlates in terms of which they may be explained. This argument is based on the logical possibility of a physiological reductionism and not on the discovery of it. It thus constitutes an article of faith about the prospects of scientific progress rather than an appeal to presently available evidence. It must be regarded therefore, as merely a hope that psychiatry will someday be comfortably claimed as medicine's own. However dim or bright the prospects for this may be, it cannot be cashed in at this early date as the justification for the use of the medical model in psychiatry.

The very search for the physiological basis of behavior should prompt the questions: Whose behavior will be searched for a physiological explanation? And why, for what purposes? Mental illness is identified exclusively by means of social and ethical (normative) criteria and not on the basis of medical (physiological) tests or standards. There is therefore no more reason to assume that the behavior of persons to whom this label is given is determined by physiological factors than there is to assume that criminal or immoral behaviors are so determined. And there is no less reason to assume that noble or virtuous acts are not physiologically determined. There is yet no basis for the belief that biochemical systems become deranged according to predominant social customs or the values of powerful men. Yet, there is a belief among psychiatrists that only the behavior of individuals labelled by them as mentally ill is subject to the determining influences of physiological events.

It is justifiable to suspect that the current psychiatric search for biophysical causes of mental illness serves a social purpose. (This is not to say that research into the physiological correlates of behavior is not also a justified and legitimate subject of scientific inquiry.) By regarding only those persons whom we diagnose as mentally ill as if their behavior has been determined by disorders of their brain tissue, we may treat them as if their behavior is caused rather than purposive; we may treat them as if they are victims rather than wrongdoers. This justifies our "treating" these persons against their will. It justifies our stripping them of the responsibility for their actions and, under the guise of medical treatment, confining them and coercively manipulating their thoughts and actions. Whether or not this is proper is an ethical and political matter. The hope of psychiatrists, however, that the use of the medical model will someday be vindicated by the discovery of twisted brain molecules may be interpreted as in the service of their primary function of controlling and altering behavior, rather than of understanding it.

Medical Physicians and Psychiatrists Are Similar Because They Perform Similar Diagnostic Functions

The proponents of the medical model in psychiatry correctly maintain that some persons who have problems in their lives, but who have no organic disease, complain of symptoms similar to persons who do have organic disease.

The reverse is also true, namely that persons with physical disease may complain of subjective experiences similar to those of persons with disturbing problems in their lives.

It is argued that since psychiatrists are sometimes called upon to determine whether an individual suffers from physical or mental illness, and since the diagnosis of diseases of the body is a medical function, psychiatrists perform functions similar to those of medical physicians. Consequently they must be viewed according to the medical model, as physicians.

This argument is rich in facts but poor in logic. It is true that individuals seen by psychiatrists sometimes have physical diseases and sometimes do not and that it is the function of the physician to tell the difference. It is also true that the psychiatrist is also a physician and may diagnose medical illness in his patients. This, however, does not imply that everything the psychiatrist does is medical in nature and should be viewed according to the medical model.

The fact that a man is a physician and sometimes performs tasks similar in every respect to those of other physicians does not mean that he cannot also perform nonmedical tasks, which must be understood in terms of some other model than the medical one. Physicians may also play golf, join political parties, and become a parent. They can also give advice on matters of conduct, promote changes in the behavior of deviant persons, and help to acquaint an individual with his biography and style of life. The fact that a person carries the credentials of a physician does not stamp his every function as medical in nature.

Also, the fact that psychiatrists are physicians and may perform medical functions does not imply that they must or ought to perform these functions. A person's medical illness may influence his behavior in a number of respects. However, not all persons who deal with him must be physicians who function to determine which features of his behavior are influenced by his disease. For instance, one of the reasons for an athlete's losing a contest or performing poorly may be a debilitating physical condition. The possibility of his having a physical disease does not justify requiring that his coach be a physician in order to make the determination. The majority of a coach's functions require that he develop skills other than being able to distinguish between physical disease and other causes of athletic failure. It is perfectly reasonable, therefore, that he hire a physician with whom he may consult about the health of his players.

Similarly, the majority of psychiatric functions require skills and knowledge other than medical. That a patient's complaints may have an organic basis is not a compelling reason for a psychiatrist to function as a physician. The psychiatrist could do what the coach does: He could refer his patient to a medical specialist, or suggest that his patient consult with one. Most psychiatrists do this; they recognize that they do not have the skill and knowledge to perform medical diagnoses and treatments. Thus, it is possible for the psychiatrist to avoid functioning as a medical physician while still functioning as a psychiatrist. If he did this (and most psychiatrists do) there would be no basis for the argument that the medical model is applicable to psychiatry because psychiatrists function in a manner similar to other physicians.

The differentiation between a physical and a psychological basis of a complaint can be made only by performing a physical examination. Psychological skills and knowledge alone cannot be employed to include or exclude the possibility of physical disease.[21] Thus, psychiatric and medical skills are separate and distinct and it is more accurate to say that the psychiatrist-physician acquires "two skills under one skull" than it is to say that psychiatry is a medical skill. The word "psychosomatic" can no better conjoin the physical and the mental than could Descartes' pineal gland. The psychic and the somatic represent two different categories of language that are employed in association with two distinct methods of scientific investigation.[22] The so-called "psychosomaticist" actually employs these two methods and languages at different times. They are conjoined only by his single personhood and by his interest in their relationship. This does not mean that no attempts should be made to correlate the psychological and the physiological. However, the medical and the psychological approach are independent in a way that the medical and, for instance, the anatomical approach are not. Skills in anatomy are components of medical skills; the skills of psychiatry are independent additions to medical skills. Once the medical and the psychological are recognized as distinct methods of approach, there is no compelling logic that insists that they be joined together by the application of the medical model to both, although there may be compelling social reasons for doing so.

The similarity between psychiatry and medicine is not based on the fact that psychiatry is a medical practice. It is based on the insistence of psychiatrists that they sometimes should perform medical functions rather than consult medical physicians. This insistence is not the *result* of a similarity between what medical doctors do and what psychiatrists do. It is one *cause* of such similarity. What is purported to be a similarity between medical and psychiatric operations is actually no more than the performance by psychiatrists of medical operations. The fact that psychiatrists do sometimes perform medical functions is not an adequate justification for conceptualizing their nonmedical functions according to the medical model.

Medical Doctors and Psychiatrists Are Similar Because They Use Similar Forms of Treatment

A fourth argument maintains that since psychiatrists use drugs and physical treatments, from the *practical* point of view they must be physicians and from the *conceptual* point of view their functions ought to be explained in terms of the medical model.

It is true that, in certain cases, psychiatrists prescribe and administer drugs and such physical treatments as shock therapy. It is probably also true that these treatments are most safely administered under the supervision of a physician. However, the fact that the technique or means of treatment is medical in nature does not mean that the purpose and effects of the treatment are medical or that the entire procedure must be conceptualized according to the medical model. Drugs and shock therapies undeniably have physiological effects on the recipients and these effects may be understood in physiological and medical terms. Drugs and physical manipulations of individuals, however, may also have social purposes, consequences, and implications, and these ought to be conceptualized in social rather than medical terms.

There are important differences between the purposes of medical and psychiatric treatment. The purpose of medical treatment is to alter the structure and function of the body to influence favorably the course of a physical disease. The purpose of psychiatric treatment is to alter mood, thought, and behavior. To use an unhappy analogy, disease-producing organisms are used in medicine to immunize by innoculation. Disease-producing organisms may also be used in bacterial warfare for the destruction of troops or population. It does not follow that since these organisms are used in both cases that bacterial warfare is a medical activity. By similar reasoning, it does not follow that because drugs are used by both medical physicians and psychiatrists that psychiatry is a medical activity.

Nor can it be argued that the physical manipulation of one person by another must necessarily be construed as a medical activity. Psychiatrists give shock treatments to alter a person's mood, thought, and behavior. Parents may whip their children for the same purpose, but we do not consider this to be a medical activity. Brainwashing, as we learned during the Korean War, may involve the physical manipulation of the prisoner by depriving him of water, food, and sleep, by exposing him to excessive heat or cold, and even by administering drugs to him. Brainwashing, however, is considered to be not a medical activity but a political one.

Physicians (or other specialists in the use of drugs) probably administered drugs to the victims of communist brainwashing in the North Korean and Chinese prisoner of war camps.[23]

In these cases, it is clear that physicians are simply technicians whose skills are used for social and political purposes. The means are medical, but the ends are social and political. The fact that psychiatrists are also physicians permits them to use themselves as the medical technicians for psychiatric ends. These ends are also social and political, rather than medical; they involve manipulating and controlling an individual's mood, thought, and behavior. By using the rhetoric of the means to describe the entire procedure, psychiatrists disguise drug administration as a medical activity. Even if it is granted that physicians are required to administer drugs to psychiatric "patients" the purpose of this activity need not be conceptualized in terms of the medical model.

It is also important to recognize that the drug-administering physician's knowledge of physiology and pharmacology serve different functions in medicine and psychiatry. The medical physician requires this knowledge to select properly the drug that will cure his patient's bodily disease. The psychiatrist requires this knowledge to avoid causing bodily damage to his patient in the course of altering his mood, thought, or actions.

We must be alert to the language used to describe the drugs and manipulations employed by psychiatrists. The fact that the substances they use are called "drugs" does not mean that they cannot be used for social purposes. Alcohol, for example, is a drug used socially. Although at times it may be medicinally prescribed, it is not considered to be a medicine. The bartenders who dispense it are not required to be doctors, nor are the merchants who retail it required to be druggists. This was not always true.

During Prohibition, alcohol was defined by law as a medicine that could be used legally only with a doctor's prescription. This is true today for psychiatric drugs. A wide variety of substances, for instance, barbiturates, tranquilizers, antidepressants (pep pills), marihuana, LSD and opium are used for social purposes—to create dreamlike states, to induce euphoria, to stimulate colorful and unusual perceptions, and so on. The laws that prohibit the use of these drugs are not based on their medical nature. Quite the contrary, the selection of these drugs for regulation affirms the fact of a nonmedical use for them.

The question of whether a drug will be defined as a medicine and restricted to medical use, or defined as a substance that may be used for social purposes depends on social and economic factors. For instance, the use of drugs to relieve depression is considered to be medical. Once a person's mood has been elevated to an optimum, any further use of that drug to create euphoria is considered to be social and is prohibited by law. The use of tranquilizing substances is considered to be medical if an individual is agitated and disturbing. The medical use ends when he is calmed. The further use of the drug to create a carefree apathy is considered to be nonmedical and is legally punishable.[24]

These definitions depend on considering excessive elation and excessive apathy to be "diseases": to be deviant behavior that must be modified toward the social norm. We are a production, consumption, and achievement oriented society with puritanical roots. Pleasure and self-indulgence are considered to be sins; hard work, economic productivity, and social moderation are considered to be virtues. Psychiatric definitions of disease reflect these normative values. When a chemical agent leads to the violation of these norms, we call the use of it "social" and prohibit it. When a chemical agent leads from the violation of these norms to conformity with them, we call the use of it medical and permit psychiatrists to use it.

The argument that the medical model is applicable to psychiatry because both psychiatrists and medical doctors use similar forms of treatment is circuitous. It depends on defining the drugs and physical "treatments" used by psychiatrists as medical in nature; and this depends on defining the persons with whom psychiatrists deal as ill. Almost all of the drugs and physical manipulations used by psychiatrists could be employed for social purposes—to influence thought, feeling, and conduct. This is true for relatively few of the drugs used by medical physicians; it applies primarily to narcotics and other drugs and procedures that reduce pain.

Far from being a support for the use of the medical model in psychiatry, the similarity in the forms of treatment used by psychiatrists and medical physicians is largely a consequence of the use of that model to define psychiatric interventions as medical in nature. The utility of the medical model is not to explain psychiatric activities, but to disguise them in the rhetoric of medicine.

THE DEFINITION OF DISEASE IN TERMS OF THE STRUCTURE AND FUNCTION OF THE BODY IS TOO NARROW AND SHOULD BE EXPANDED TO INCLUDE OTHER DIMENSIONS OF HUMAN EXISTENCE

According to this argument the traditional view that disease refers to an undesirable alteration in bodily structure and function has become obsolete. The term "disease" can no longer be limited to bodily events, nor even to a state of the individual. The term must be expanded to include the various dimensions of human existence—the psychological, social, political, and even the spiritual dimensions of life.[25] This argument does not maintain that these other dimensions should be reduced to a material basis, but rather that the concept of disease ought to be applied to the total range of human experience.

This argument does not depend on the discovery of new facts about disease; it is a plea for the redefinition of the term. Instead of referring to the bodily state of an individual, the term "disease," it is maintained, should refer to the broader problems of Good and Evil—problems mankind is concerned with solving—poverty, illiteracy, crime, delinquency, the crises of the life cycle, and war.

The redefinition of disease in psychiatry is not a new phenomenon. It is the hallmark of psychiatric revolutions. When the concept of illness was stretched beyond its application to bodily disorders to include "disorders" of human behavior, it was only a matter of time before it encompassed the entire human drama. Then it became necessary for psychiatric theory to take into account what philosophers and social scientists have known since, at least, the time of the Enlightenment—that human conduct is also social in nature and is the product of shared history, culture, and aspirations and of the creative choice of individuals.

What were psychiatrists to do when they finally recognized that to understand and alter "mental illness" they must understand and alter psychological, behavioral, social, economic, cultural, and political events instead of physical, biochemical, and physiological ones? This created a crisis in psychiatric identity that could be met with one of two solutions. First, psychiatrists could have frankly admitted that the methods, language, and conceptual models of medicine were poorly suited to the understanding of man in culture. They could have conceded that the medical model was deficient as a scientific model because it concealed important differences between the language of physics and the language of psychology, between the body and behavior, and between the activities of medical physicians and those of psychiatrists. They could have abandoned the medical model for the conceptual models of the social sciences. The term "disease" would then retain its paradigmatic use to refer to disorders of bodily structure and function. "Disorders" of personal behavior and social organization would retain their own distinctive, ordinary language names, or new, nonmedical names for them could be coined.

The consequences of this course of action would be to weaken or to sever the ties between psychiatry and medicine and to create new bonds between psychiatry and the social sciences. Psychiatry, however, was deeply imbedded in medicine not only conceptually but also socially and institutionally.

Such a separation could not be easily accomplished. Moreover, there were strong social pressures for continuing the alliance between psychiatry and medicine because of the socially valuable services performed by psychiatrists under the rubric of medical treatment. Also, the separation of psychiatry and medicine would have given equal title to psychologists, sociologists, anthropologists, and others to conduct therapy and to administer the social programs of psychiatry. This would have weakened the authority of psychiatrists, and, hence, been to their disadvantage.

The second path is the one chosen by modern psychiatry. Instead of rejecting the medical model of disease as inadequate to their new social knowledge and social programs, and instead of redefining psychiatry as a nonmedical enterprise, they enlarged the concept of disease and the boundaries of medicine to include the total relationship of the individual to his society. This change was not simply a matter, as some suggested,[26] of recognizing that man as an organism could not be understood independently of his environment. Physicians have understood this principle well since the time of Darwin. The enlargement of the concept of disease and the scope of medicine *declared* that the relationship of the individual and his society was the proper arena for psychiatric study and intervention. It made the concepts of medical psychiatry compatible with the expanding activities of psychiatrists outside the traditional areas of medicine.

Once they broadened their concerns to include all dimensions of human behavior, psychiatrists began to find the concept of disease unwieldy and began to modify or abandon it. They now speak instead of crises, problems in living, maladaptation, maladjustment, personal troubles, and social disturbances. However, this hedging will not do. Much hinges on whether or not the problems with which psychiatrists deal are diseases. For instance, if they are not diseases, then what is the justification for the involuntary "hospitalization" of large numbers of persons in the name of their mental health?

This broadening of the medical model so that the concept of disease includes all manner of social problems and social suffering suggests that the use of the medical model in psychiatry is strained and contrived. It can be employed only by the most radical redefinition of medicine, so that psychiatry can maintain its medical identity while it becomes involved in all dimensions of social and political life. The broadening of the concept of disease is not an argument for the use of the medical model in psychiatry. It is a device for perpetuating that use.

THE MEDICAL MODEL IN PSYCHIATRY:
IDEA OR IDEOLOGY?

There are, it is true, certain similarities between psychiatry and medicine. Some of these similarities, however, are superficial and are based only on a common medical rhetoric. Other similarities are actually overlaps in function. They result from psychiatrists performing medical functions such as physical examinations and the treatment of such medical illnesses as organic brain disease.

The differences between medical and psychiatric situations and operations are profound. The idea that psychiatry is different from medicine is not novel. It is expressed in the often heard complaint of psychiatrists that their medical training was of little value in preparing them for their eventual functions. (This is not quite true. Their medical training is of little instrumental value, but it is of immense social value in establishing an identity base from which to undertake their operations.) It is expressed by the scepticism of the patronizing internist who confidentially hints that he does not regard his psychiatric colleagues to be *really* doctors or to *really* practice medicine; nor does he regard their patients to be *really* sick. That the psychiatrist, in turn, regards this internist as naive, behind the times, and in need of some "mental health education" further emphasizes the differences between psychiatry and medicine. No other group of medical specialists spends quite the amount of time and energy that psychiatrists do in denying that they are a separate breed or in attempting to persuade their brethren-in-credentials that they are kin under the sheepskin.

The use of the medical model in psychiatry serves to emphasize the similarities between medicine and psychiatry and to obscure their differences. It functions therefore, not so much to clarify and explain the nature of psychiatry as to persuade us to view it in a certain way—as a medical science and practice that deals with mental illness.

The medical model ignores or disguises distinctive features of psychiatric situations; this suggests that it functions as an ideology. Karl Mannheim[27] developed the concept of ideology in an attempt to formulate the relationship between ideas and social interests. According to Mannheim, the concept of ideology reflects the fact that individuals or groups may become so intensely interest-bound to a situation that their thinking reflects facts that serve that interest and ignores facts that would undermine it. The contrasting concept is that of utopia, which reflects the fact that individuals or groups interested in change will in their thinking, reflect facts favorable to that change and ignore facts that might obstruct it. Although Mannheim's concepts developed from his study of political conflict, they have broader application to any ideas that obscure actual circumstances in the service of social interests.

Mannheim distinguished "particular" from "total" ideologies. By "particular ideology," Mannheim referred to:

> . . . all those utterances the "falsity" of which is due to an intentional or unintentional, conscious, semi-conscious, or unconscious deluding of one's self or of others, taking place on a psychological level and structurally resembling lies . . . [They are] specific assertions which may be regarded as concealments, falsifications or lies without attacking the integrity of the *total mental structure* of the asserting subjects.[28]

Thus, the medical model of psychiatry may be viewed as a particular ideology, as a concealment of the differences between medical and psychiatric operations, and therefore, a concealment of the social nature of psychiatry to promote particular social functions and social interests. The exact nature of these functions and interests can only be explicated by a full description of the social functions of psychiatry.

To assert that the concept of mental illness is a particular ideology does not impeach other aspects of the conceptual structure of psychiatry, although other concepts may also be analyzed as particular ideologies. Thus, the science of psychiatry may contain statements that pass empirical tests even though other statements may be ideological.

The concept of "total" ideology is roughly equivalent to the sociology of knowledge. The theory of the sociology of knowledge concerns itself with the role of extra-theoretical factors in developing thought. It deals with the influence of social settings, social processes, and the collective purposes of a group on the modes and content of the thought of that group. While the study of "particular" ideologies implies an effort to ". . . unmask the more or less conscious deceptions and disguises of human interest groups . . . ,"[29] the study of "total" ideologies implies an effort to understand the character of thought in terms of the different social and historical settings in which it occurs.

An exhaustive study of psychiatric thought thus must include two separate inquiries, neither of which has been adequately undertaken for reasons profoundly related to the ideological nature of the medical model in psychiatry and to the sociopolitical nature of psychiatry as a social institution. First, it requires the study of psychiatric thought and rhetoric as particular ideologies, as socially useful deceptions. It is especially necessary to scrutinize the medical model in psychiatry as a particular ideology because this model has been most responsible for the association of psychiatry with medicine and the consequent shielding of psychiatry from the critical examination of social thinkers.

Second, it requires that psychiatric thought and the practices that are based on and justified by that thought be related to the social and historical fabric of Western culture. It requires a search that penetrates beyond the character of psychiatry as a medical science and practice, to its nature as an historical movement, which, like all such movements, must be understood in the context of social, economic, and political process and change.

CHAPTER THREE

The Social Matrix of Medicine

. . . medicine is not so much a natural as a social science. The goal of medicine is social. It is not only the cure of disease, the restoration of an organism. The goal is to keep man adjusted to his environment as a useful member of society or to readjust him as the case may be.

—HENRY SIGERIST[1]

Now when we speak of health or disease, we use certain implicit values. Health is something good and desirable, while disease, whatever else it means, implies something bad.

—LESTER KING[2]

To understand the meaning and function of the medical model, and thus to understand the application of that model to the psychiatric situation, it is necessary to consider its use in medicine.

Medicine is a social activity, as is any activity of a shared or sharable nature. Yet, there is a tendency to think of medicine as above culture, politics, and beliefs—as rooted in the "scientific" structure of the world rather than in human designs and purposes. Thus, there is a tendency to think that the character of medical practice is determined primarily by scientific research and instrumentation, even in an age of socialized medicine.

According to this view, medicine consists of applying scientific knowledge to the maintenance and repair of the human body. Medical concepts, such as health and disease, are therefore thought to be similar to other scientific concepts, for instance of positive and negative charge in electromagnetics. The difficulty of defining the vague concepts of health and disease is attributed to the paucity of our scientific knowledge rather than to their permeation with social values.

Nevertheless, the goals of medicine are social and moral. They are not the product of scientific research but of the striving of human beings to intervene in their own destinies. The relationship of individuals to the healers of their bodies is a complex social arrangement permeated with all the trappings of modern life. Hygienic practices are woven into the cultural fabric. The social dimensions of health practices become increasingly difficult to recognize in a society in which the use of scientific technology is rapidly increasing. The cloak of science, however, cannot disguise the body of culture to the observer who looks with anthropological vision.[3]

THE SOCIAL MATRIX OF MEDICAL SCIENCE

The social matrix of medical *practice* is much more obvious than is the social matrix of medical *science*. Modern conceptions of medical science are influenced by the idea that physical science is value neutral, that it is independent of human aspirations, motivations, political interests, and social processes. The quest for knowledge, however, is a fully socialized act. Scientific inquiry is nurtured by yesterday's unanswered questions, assumes the character of today's customs, techniques and resources, and presses into a tomorrow it will help to shape.

Medical scientists should need no reminder of the ethical

context of their endeavors. The goals of medical science may be selected and approved or avoided and condemned. No matter how "pure" the research, no matter how distant from the possibility of beneficial application, the constant, underlying goal of medical researchers is that the results of their labor will alleviate human suffering.[4] Even if humanistic motives are denied in favor of the "disinterested," "objective" search for scientific truth, medical researchers must recognize the presence of social and ethical issues at three distinct points in their work: (1) in the selection of a subject for study, which is influenced by such factors as patterns of funding, availability of facilities and sponsors, disciplinary faddism, career ambitions, and the urgency of certain problems; (2) in the selection of research designs and techniques which are governed by moral and legal codes; and (3) in the practical uses of medical research, which often depends on weighing the desirable and undesirable aspects of a procedure.

Human values have an even more profound relevance to medical science than is indicated by these three factors, a relevance that has deep significance for medicine and an even greater significance for psychiatry. To understand the social and ethical matrix of medicine it is necessary to examine the nature of health and disease. These concepts are not scientific categories, but are based on values that define certain human conditions as bad and to be avoided and others as desirable and to be pursued. These values are rooted in the passionate human desire for a long life free of pain and disability. They are also rooted in that highly developed human purposefulness by which man employs his environment to intervene in the course of his natural destiny.

THE CONCEPTS OF HEALTH AND DISEASE

What is Disease?

How do medical scientists distinguish between health and disease? The question posed here goes beyond an inquiry into the nature of specific diseases and diagnostic criteria. The question is not "What is pneumonia or cirrhosis?" but is "What is the meaning of the word 'disease'?" This question is seldom posed, yet it is so important that it is helpful to put it in hypothetical form. Let us imagine a Master Physiologist with a complete knowledge of the workings of the human body, including all variations under all earthly conditions, but no knowledge of which of these variations is to be labelled as diseased and which as healthy. How can he decide what is disease?

He could not decide this question by attempting to discover the normal and the abnormal because these are not qualities that may be discovered by examining and analyzing the structure and function of the body. They are ascribed to bodily states and are themselves neither tissues nor processes. Furthermore, the qualities of normality and abnormality presuppose precisely the distinction we are seeking.

Perhaps he could employ statistical techniques to determine which bodily states occur most frequently and which most seldom (statistical normality). A statistical distribution of bodily phenomena, however, is not an adequate criterion for distinguishing disease from health. After he had obtained a full tabulation of the frequency with which all bodily states occur in a large population, he would be left with the problem of specifying some demarcation point that would separate diseased from healthy states. Furthermore, how would he know whether disease is the more or less frequently occurring variation? Certain diseases occur with great frequency, for instance when they are endemic to a particular area or during an epidemic. Others occur rarely. Also, false symptoms of disease may occur under special circumstances, for instance, an individual may have a temperature elevation to 101° either because he has been exercising on a hot day or because he has an infection.[5]

Let us suppose, however, that our Master Physiologist discovered that a particular bodily event, for instance the occlusion of an artery to the heart muscle, was regularly associated with death, pain, or disability. In a universe free of human purpose and valuation, such a regularity would be a fact without significance, a mere instance of the continuous and endless process of the change and metamorphosis of matter. However, to a human being who has the capacity to sense his own mortality, to anticipate and fear death, suffering, and helplessness, such a regularity has the greatest significance. The desire to avoid or at least delay these catastrophes leads us to search for points at which we may intervene in natural processes in the service of life and well-being. Our desire to intervene in bodily processes in order to achieve a long life, free of pain and disability is the basis for the identification of disease and the distinction of it from health.

Health and disease are neither structures nor functions of the body as are, for instance, the heart and the circulation. They cannot be discovered and investigated in the same way as can a nerve tract or a hormone. "Health" and "disease" are *labels* used to classify and denote bodily states in medicine, but they themselves are not bodily states. Diseases, unlike material objects, do not exist independently of the purpose and designs of scientists. Instead of asking "what are 'health' and 'disease'?" therefore, it is more appropriate to inquire into their meaning: to inquire into the situation and purposes for which these terms are used.

The primary meanings of the terms "health" and "disease" are ethical; they are designs for action.[6] Those states denoted by the term "health" are considered to be desirable and to require action designed for their maintenance. Other states, denoted by the term "disease" are considered to be undesirable and are to be eliminated, forestalled, or prevented. In medical practice, the term "disease" may be replaced by "undesirable" and the term "health" by "desirable." The importance of this for psychiatry cannot be overstressed.

Once a bodily state has been classified as a disease (as undesirable), scientific methods may be employed to investigate its natural history—its causes, its course, its connections, and its presence or absence in a particular individual. These methods include statistical surveys, clinical observations, and biochemical and pathological studies. This information increases our knowledge about the workings of the body under conditions we label "diseased." But the question of whether a bodily state is to be classified as a disease at all is not, strictly speaking, a scientific matter. It depends on whether we consider that state to be desirable or whether we associate it with the undesirable experiences of pain, disability, and death.

Disease as the Focus of Medical Intervention

To classify as diseases bodily states that we did not wish to eliminate but simply wished to categorize for scientific purposes would be absurd. Nor would it be sensible to classify as healthy, states that we consider undesirable and in whose natural course we intend to intervene. The categories of health and disease are not abstract scientific concepts devised to enlighten our understanding. The main motive for classifying certain bodily states as diseased and others as healthy is to intervene in the course of bodily processes to eliminate or to preserve them.

Intervention is central to the meaning of the terms "health" and "disease." It is the pivot about which medical practice and medical science swing. To understand medicine it is necessary to understand the rules and aims of medical intervention. These rules are, in part, determined by the anatomical and physiological characteristics of the body, the properties of drugs, and the possibilities of such physical manipulations as surgery. Learning the rules of these interventions is the primary task of the medical student. There is no reason, however, to limit a consideration of the rules of medical intervention to their scientific and technical aspects. The rules or ethics of medical intervention are also social in nature and are deeply rooted in the ecological, ideological, social, and political character of a people.

The broadest and most complete views of disease and

medical practice must include the context of culture as well as of physicochemical events.[7] Even the idea that disease is a scientifically determined concept and that medical interventions are determined purely by technical considerations is culture bound. It is characteristic of differentiated societies in which entities are abstracted from experience and in which human actions are viewed in the nonmoral context of science and technology.

Disease and the Abstraction of Medical Science

The abstraction of the idea of disease from the context of social life and human values probably began at the dawn of recorded history, with the beginning of a specialized and serious interest in abstract speculation, in truth for its own sake. As a special class of philosopher-scientist developed, the pursuit of knowledge became differentiated from social regulatory functions and, to a degree, from the practical aspects of life.

During the Renaissance, a vigorous interest developed in the scientific study of man, an important part of which was the study of the human body as a magnificent biophysical machine. As biophysical science and technology developed in logarithmic leaps and bounds, a more refined appreciation of the structure and function of the human body was gained. Diseases that were previously thought to be single entities were separated into their various components, and causes were distinguished from symptoms. For instance, it became known that dropsy, a deadly swelling of the body, is not a disease in itself, but is a symptom of kidney, liver, heart, or malnutritional disease. In the spirit of nineteenth-century biology, a huge list of diseases were classified and systematized, including many which had not undesirable effects, but which were structurally or functionally similar to those that did.

Gradually, a new breed of physician developed whose main function was not to heal but to conduct research. Thus, advances in medical knowledge often took place outside of the practical context of medical intervention, in the more purely intellectual surroundings of the laboratory. Diseases were given a scientific life of their own on the basis of some systematic similarity to other pathology, rather than on the basis of that call for medical intervention from which their status had always emanated. Medical science became a rationalized and abstracted structure that tended to ignore and obscure the social and ethical foundations on which it stood.

It is worthwhile to consider in some detail the concepts of homeostasis, adaptation, and adjustment. These concepts illustrate the manner in which modern medical thought may obscure the social matrix of health and disease. These concepts are also relevant because they are sometimes used as evidence of a theoretical relationship between medicine and psychiatry.

According to these concepts, living systems are in dynamic equilibrium with their environment. Homeostasis refers to ". . . the process whereby the internal environment fluctuates within fairly narrow limits as the result of reactions to disturbances induced from within or without."[8] Adaptation refers to the particular responses of an organism that enable it to remove a stimulus for behavior.[9] So long as pressures toward change are satisfactorily balanced by countervailing measures, a steady state is achieved and life continues. If, however, the stimulus upsets the homeostatic equilibrium, it is considered to be a stress that may result in disease or death. Health consists of the successful maintenance of homeostasis or adaptation to stress; disease consists of the unsuccessful adaptation to stress.

These concepts are held to provide a basis for a unified theory of health and disease. First, they are considered to provide a theoretical unification of biological life at all levels because all organisms in the evolutionary scale demonstrate homeostasis, adaptation, and adjustment. Second, they are considered to be the basis of a unitary theory of physical and mental health because it is assumed that adaptation of behavior to the social environment is a process similar to the adaptation of the body to the physical environment.

Let us grant that life is sustained only within a certain range of variability and that the discovery of this fact was an important advance in science. What is the relevance of this fact to the concepts of health and disease? There are essentially two possibilities.

First, it is possible that the discovery of the homeostatic nature of life is a new fact that may be *correlated* positively with the occurrence of health and negatively with disease. If this is correct, it should be possible, in principle, to conceive of a failure in homeostasis independently of the presence or absence of disease. Conversely, it should be possible, in principle, to imagine disease or death in the circumstance of perfect homeostasis, adjustment, or adaptation. For if the processes of homeostasis, adaptation, and adjustment can be correlated with disease and death the two types of events must be independently identifiable.

What would it mean, however, to say that a man is prostrate and moribund but that his body remains in perfect homeostasis? The set of facts by which disease and death are identified are identical with the set of facts by which a failure of homeostasis, adaptation, or adjustment are identified. In other words, the presence of disease is the criterion used to determine that a failure of homeostasis or adaptation has occurred.

This means the second possibility is more likely, namely, that the terms "homeostasis," "adaptation," and "adjustment" are refined restatements at a higher level of abstraction of the term "health." The failure of "homeostasis," "adaptation," and "adjustment" represent refined restatements at a higher level of abstraction of the term "disease." At the heart of the matter is the idea that the terms "success" and "failure" of homeostasis introduce the same ethical variables contained in the meaning of the words "health" and "disease." Successful adaptation logically *implies* a state of health; a failure of adaptation *logically implies* a state of disease or death. Since the concept of the failure of homeostasis is definitionally (or tautologically) related to the idea of disease, failure of homeostasis cannot constitute a causal explanation of disease and death.

The same type of analysis can be made of the concept of stress as a cause of disease. Once the presence of a disease is recognized we label the cause of that disease as a stress. Stress, however, does not cause pneumonia; bacteria do. Nevertheless, bacteria may be *defined* as stressful agents. This is because stresses are defined by their effects. If a stimulus may cause pain, disability, or death, it is defined as a stress. Stress, therefore, cannot be the cause of disease since it is definitionally related to it.

The concepts of stress, adaptation, homeostasis, and adjustments belong to a higher level of abstraction than the particular physiological and behavioral events they denote. Their use is therefore an example of the manner in which abstract terms tend to assume a concrete meaning in modern science.

Two important and relevant consequences result from the concrete use of these abstract terms in medicine and psychiatry.

Terms Become Less Specific

These terms accomplish what all abstractions accomplish: They eliminate specific actions and events from the context of thought. At the same time, these terms give the impression that they refer to events in the world, the knowledge of which is independent of the actions and judgments of men. For instance, terms such as "the failure of homeostasis" are often used to give the impression that what is being referred to is a natural event, which would occur whether or not it was being observed. A failure, of whatever kind, however, is a judgment about an event rather than an event itself. "A failure of homeostasis," therefore, is not an event, but is a manner of conceptualizing and evaluating an event; it is an ascribed rather than a described quality. These abstract terms are a step away from the operational philosophy that is characteristic of modern physics.[10] They tend to distract from the fact that knowledge about natural and social events is gained transactionally rather than passively.[11]

Terms Disguise Social and Ethical Matrix

The concepts of homeostasis, adaptation, and adjustment acknowledge the dynamic nature of life. They disguise, however, the values placed on the quality and direction of change. They thus disguise the social and ethical matrix of medicine and psychiatry. To say about a man's behavior only that it is maladaptive or maladjusted, is to ignore the specific nature and context of his actions, their social and ethical significance and the "politics" that underlie the disapproval of them. In the context of social behavior, homeostasis, adjustment, or adaptation may imply conformity with prevailing social rules or powerful figures, and the failure of homeostasis, adjustment or adaptation may indicate rebellion, criminality or conflict with a powerful social interest. By distracting from the social and ethical matrix of judgments of failure and success, these concepts seem to achieve the status of objective, value-neutral scientific concepts. They thus lend themselves to use as "scientifically authoritative" statements justifying social evaluations and actions. Finally, by referring both to human and animal life and by claiming to provide a unified theory of mental and physical health and disease, these terms emphasize the similarities rather than the differences between medicine and psychiatry. By so doing, they contribute to the particular ideology of psychiatry that serves to disguise its social and ethical functions. Thus, these terms surreptitiously acquire the political significance they were designed to avoid.

Disease and the Technicalization and
Bureaucratization of Medical Practice

Recent changes in scientific technology and social organization have helped divorce the concepts of health and disease from the social context of medical practice. Advances in scientific technology have resulted in the refinement of diagnostic procedures so that the decision for medical intervention seems more often to be made by the physician, on the basis of his interpretation of the medical facts, than by the patient on the basis of a call for relief from his symptoms. Changes in social organization have interposed into the physician-patient relationship, powerful third parties who often tend to impose their own rules on the medical transaction. The effect of these two changes is to shift the control of medical intervention away from the patient toward the medical expert and the bureaucracy and to imbue the concept of disease with an abstract and technical connotation.

The information and instrument explosion of the past three decades has greatly expanded and prolonged the process of medical education. As medical science and technology have become more differentiated, physicians have tended to specialize. With specialization the physician's focus narrows to body parts and functions. Whenever man is reduced to his component parts, the effect is to diminish ethical sensitivities toward him, since the unit of ethical perception is the social person, rather than any of his physical parts. As diagnostic and therapeutic practices become increasingly complex and numerous, and as medical emphasis is placed on prevention, early detection, and the diagnosis of exotic and subclinical entities, the physician becomes more task oriented than patient oriented.

As a result, the physician tends to view disease as a fixed entity, diagnosed and treated by following established routines and procedures, instead of as a deeply human call for relief from pain, disability, and the prospect of death. The patient becomes an object to be acted on, rather than a "property owner" who (owns his body and) has certain rights and privileges. This tends to shift the concepts of health and disease away from the valuation of life and well-being toward the technical advice of a health expert who must be relied on to determine the desirability of medical intervention.

Within the past hundred years, an increasing number of

social institutions have become participants in the doctor-patient relationship: government, business, the schools, the military, insurance companies, and so on. One of the most important institutional additions to medical practice, as in all of the "tinkering trades," is the "workshop complex"—the hospital.[12]

As medical techniques have become more complicated and sophisticated, medical practice is increasingly conducted in a hospital and laboratory setting. Hospitals are technocracies within bureaucracies, and hospital personnel are organized along classic bureaucratic lines.[13] The experiences of the hospitalized patient are determined by bureaucratic rules and technical procedures. The patient often feels that he is merely an object to be serviced, that he is expected to commend his fate into the hands of the officials and experts with whose almost mystical recommendations and orders he is expected to comply.

The interposition of any third party imbues the doctor-patient relationship with bureaucratic qualities. When these agencies pay the piper, they acquire the power to call the orchestration, if not the tune. The larger, more powerful, and more differentiated the third party, the greater the routinization and impersonality of medical intervention will be and the more the practice of medicine becomes that—

> . . . wonderful brand of "non-person treatment" found in the medical world, whereby the patient is greeted with what passes as civility, and said farewell to in the same fashion, with everything in between going on as if the patient weren't there as a social person at all, but only as a possession someone has left behind.[14]

One need only compare the social situations of the draft board physical examination, the military sick call, the charity clinic, and the charity hospital ward to the situation of the plush private hospital suite and the private office practice to appreciate the impact of third parties on the practice of medicine.

Technicalization and bureaucratization of modern medical practice have improved the quality and efficiency of medical care. They have, however, also served to shift attention away from the socioethical matrix of health and disease. They tend to make these concepts more abstract: to remove them from social judgments and evaluations and to give them an independent "scientific" status. They tend to transform the physician into a quasi-official scientist whose decisions and recommendations are given the authentic stamp of scientific knowledge, technical expertise, and official authority. The patient, under these circumstances, becomes an object acted on by the natural ravages of disease on the one side, and the routine, impersonal ministrations of the medical tinkering trades on the other. These social conditions tend to create the impression that the final authority for the desirability of medical intervention comes from the physician rather than from the patient, and that it is exclusively a medical and scientific determination, rather than one that is also social, ethical, and legal.

THE ETHICS OF MEDICAL INTERVENTION

Although modern medical science and practice have become abstract and bureaucratized, social, moral, and legal rules govern the call for medical intervention. Viewing the concepts of "health" and "disease" as designs for intervention requires a consideration of these rules.

A consideration of the social mechanisms by which the desirability of medical treatment is determined unavoidably leads to a consideration of social power in the doctor-patient relationship. There are two routes for initiating medical treatment: (1) The individual patient may have the power to define himself as ill and to call for medical intervention; (2) The physician, some other person, or a group may have the power to define an individual as sick and in need of medical intervention.

Patient Initiates

Two conditions enable the individual to initiate the call for medical intervention. First, the presence of disease must be recognizable to the individual who suffers from it.[15] The ability to recognize the presence of disease lies in large part with the natural mechanisms of the body. Certain alterations in bodily structure and function are associated with pain and other forms of suffering, from which there is a natural inclination to seek relief. Animals have an instinctive reaction to alleviate bodily discomfort. Dogs, for instance, will go on three legs to rest a broken fourth; monkeys will extract foreign bodies from their skin, and other animals will seek to alleviate fever by bathing in cold water.[16] These mechanisms also operate in man. In man there is also the capacity to recognize the symptoms (signals) of forthcoming discomfort, and there is the anticipation and fear of death, an event that may be forestalled by proper intervention. *Medicine is essentially a social extension of the body's natural defenses against pain, disability, and death.* Medicine is the socialized mobilization of efforts in behalf of the individual to relieve his suffering and preserve his life.[17]

The person who is stricken by the plague, whose flesh has been torn by a penetrating missile, or who is rendered helpless by swollen, immobile joints does not need an expert to tell him about his bodily state or to persuade him that medical intervention is necessary. On the other hand, when physicians are consulted routinely, by personal choice or by bureaucratic regulation, and when techniques of diagnosis have become so refined that diseases can be detected before their symptoms are apparent to the victim, then the expert becomes important in the call for medical intervention. The routinization and technicalization of medical practice tend to obscure the impulse behind the call for medical intervention—the individual's desire for long life free of pain and disability.

The second condition that enables the individual to initiate the call for medical intervention is for him to retain the social power to adopt or reject the sick role. To phrase this in legal terms, the right of consent must be unabridged either by the physician or by society. While the physician decides the kind of therapy to administer and how, such a voluntary patient decides whether it will be administered at all and sometimes when.

Non-Patient Initiates Intervention

The right of an individual to seek or reject medical intervention is suspended in certain circumstances. Under these circumstances, a government official, a family member, or a physician may have the power to insert an individual into the sick role.

When the social and political structure of a society favor the interests of the group over those of the individual, the call for medical intervention may be initiated by and serve the group. The patient may be forced to surrender his right to determine for himself the desirability of medical intervention, and the physician may function as a representative of group interests rather than as the agent of his patient. In little communities, for instance, where it may be necessary for each person to perform his tasks in the prescribed manner and not be a burden to his fellows, medicine may function as a social instrument to serve the interests of the community by intervening in its name in the life processes of an individual.

In our society, an individual's right to reject medical treatment may be suspended when it has been established that his physical condition jeopardizes public health, if, for instance, he is a typhoid carrier and refuses to submit voluntarily to treatment. This abridgment of the individual's right to determine the desirability of *medical* treatment occurs only when his *physical* condition constitutes a public health hazard. The enforced treatment is explicitly defined by law as a social action designed primarily to serve the physical health interests of the public rather than the patient.

In some medical situations the authority for treatment rests with the physician. This occurs, for instance, when the patient cannot give consent because he is unconscious or delerious and when a relative is not present to give consent for him. In such cases the physician is permitted to procede with the necessary therapeutic measures. He is, however, in a delicate legal situation. He is obliged to revert the authority for treatment to the adult patient at the earliest possible moment. As soon as the patient regains consciousness he may decide to continue or discontinue treatment or to change physicians. The physician must abide by this decision or be liable to charges of illegal assault and battery. There are other social situations in medicine in which treatment may be rendered without consent, when, for instance, the patient is a minor or when his social rights are suspended because he is a prisoner or a member of the armed forces.[18]

There are situations in medicine when an individual is deprived of his right to consent because he disagrees with his physician about the desirability of medical intervention. These situations are instructive because of the role played by the psychiatrist.

People sometimes do not desire either to seek medical treatment or to assume the social role of illness, for instance, if they are Christian Scientists. A person may not wish to be treated for a curable illness, or he may actually mutilate himself, feign illness, or attempt suicide. In these instances when an individual's valuation of health and disease differs from that of his physician or of society in general, the physician may do one of two things.

The physician may respect this person's values, no matter how idiosyncratic or self-destructive they may be, and refuse to intervene without his consent. Often, however, physicians do not interpret such idiosyncratic behavior as a dissent from the cultural consensus about the undesirability of pain, disability, and death. Instead they attempt to maintain that consensus by labelling that person as mentally ill and, in effect, disqualifying his "vote." These patients are often referred to psychiatrists who may attempt to influence them to adhere to the cultural attitudes toward health.

The instructive point is that forced treatment is accomplished by converting the medical patient into a mental patient. Such psychiatric coercion denies that a person may find value in suffering, disability, or death. This denial, however, can be accomplished only by deviating from the generally accepted *medical* practice of respecting the patient's right to withhold consent for treatment, and this denial can be accomplished only by dehumanizing the patient—by disqualifying his actions as the distorted expressions of a "sick" mind.

To seek to impose medical intervention upon an individual against his will requires forcing him into the social role of illness against his will. Thus, whatever else involuntary treatment may be, it is also social coercion. This does not mean that the person who refuses treatment does not have a condition denoted with such terms as "pneumonia" or "appendicitis"; such states exist independently of the desires of an individual for medical treatment. However, to classify certain states as diseases, and to use that classification as a basis for medical intervention without an individual's consent, is to employ an abstract, "scientific" diagnosis for the purposes of social coercion.

The fact that, in the vast majority of medical cases the patient's consent is required before the physician may procede with treatment indicates that *medicine* values the individual's sovereignty over his body. Respect for this sovereignty is directly related to the political values of a society. The right of consent is found in its purest form in societies in which the physician sells his services for a fee to patients who are free to purchase these services when and from whom they wish. The right of full consent is often abridged with the inclusion of third parties in the doctor-patient relationship. Because they usually pay the physician, these parties may acquire the power to regulate the timing of treatment, to choose the physician, and, sometimes, to insert or remove a person from the role of illness.

The political structure of the United States, in principle, fosters respect for individual rights, including the right to consent to medical treatment. Deviations from this standard, as occur in psychiatry, cannot be viewed as variations in medical practice. They must be viewed as political deviations in the direction of totalitarianism. In every country, including our own, there are pockets of totalitarianism where the individual may be coerced to surrender his sovereignty over his body to a more powerful social group—in, for instance, the armed forces, prisons, mental hospitals, certain religious orders, some universities, and even a number of business organizations.

The question of when a person suffers from a disease requiring medical intervention is thus determined by social and political factors as well as by the condition of his body. The rules of medical intervention are based on a hierarchy of values and social power. This is more apparent when powerful persons are involved, for instance, in determining the incapacity of the President and the succession of the Vice-President to power. The sociopolitical character of medical practice, however, is no less important when it concerns the average citizen. It is merely less conspicuous because medical activities are viewed as technical rather than social and ethical in nature.

THE SOCIAL CONTEXT OF MEDICINE
AS A DISGUISE FOR PSYCHIATRY

The abstraction, technicalization and routinization of modern medical practice have great significance for psychiatry. They enable psychiatrists more easily to disguise their social values and activities in the rhetoric and in the social context of medicine.

By identifying themselves as medical scientists, psychiatrists may take advantage of the popular belief that medical science is value-free and unrelated to social issues. As physicians, psychiatrists may borrow from medicine the false assumption that the distinction between health and disease is scientific rather than social and ethical. As a result, the diagnosis of a person as mentally ill is accepted as based on a purely "objective" "medical" examination of his brain, mind, and behavior rather than on a moral judgment of his social performance.

The technicalization of medical practice permits psychiatrists to suffuse their operations with the aura of medical competence and the charisma of medical expertise. Thus, psychiatrists, like medical physicians, may make the diagnosis of mental illness without requiring the confirmation of the patient's own experiences. Just as sophisticated medical techniques may be used to diagnose a disease without the individual's being aware of his affliction, so, supposedly, sophisticated psychiatric techniques may be used to diagnose a person as mentally ill without his being aware of his "condition." This gives the psychiatric "expert" the advantage of being able to label a person as mentally ill without that person's (or anyone else's) being able to provide any evidence to the contrary. The sole "evidence" required is the psychiatrist's claim that his "expertness" (his medical credentials and his "clinical experience") enables him to make the diagnosis. This, in effect, gives the psychiatrist the power to label anyone as mentally ill.

The bureaucratization and technicalization of medical practices permit psychiatry to be practiced in an institutional setting and still retain a similarity to medicine, even though medical and psychiatric institutions perform very different functions. They allow the psychiatrist to function as an agent of the state and still maintain his medical identity. They prevent a dazzled lay audience from appreciating the ethical foundations of health and disease and the social significance of psychiatric interventions. They divert attention from the psychiatrist as a social agent and tend to purify the motives, neutralize the prejudices, and blur the social interests for which he stands.

By virtue of his association with medicine, the psychiatrist is classified with other physicians as a helper. The psychiatric situation is squeezed into a medical context. The patient is considered to be (knowingly or unknowingly) in distress and the psychiatrist is considered to be his benefactor. All of the psychiatrist's actions are *defined* as helpful to the patient, and any of the patient's actions may be identified as a manifestation of the disease for which he requires treatment. The definition of the psychiatrist as a helper obliges the patient to be trusting and compliant even though he may suffer discomfort and indignity at the psychiatrists' hands. That the medical physician is so seldom the enemy of his patient, because he respects the principle of consent, distracts us from the psychiatrist's often being the enemy of the patient. The psychiatrist is the patient's enemy when the principle of consent is not respected: when committing the patient to a psychiatric hospital, or when refusing to discharge him at his request. If the patient defines his own interests as not wishing to be defined as ill, to be thrust into the social role of illness, and to be deprived of his freedom by being forced to remain in a psychiatric institution he is entitled to perceive the psychiatrist not as his benefactor, but as his captor, not as his helper but as his adversary.[19]

By employing the medical model, the psychiatrist escapes the accusation that he is the captor or adversary of his patient. By assuming the identity of the physician, who is socially defined as a helper, the psychiatrist is able to neutralize his patients' accusations. This psychiatric deception is facilitated by stretching two medical contexts in which it is permissible to treat a person against his will—when the patient is unconscious or delerious, and when the patient is a child.

It is true, of course, that the unconscious patient is not capable of giving consent for treatment. Similarly, the severely delerious patient is unable to understand a request for his consent and is, hence, unable to give it. The psychiatrist often justifies treating a person against his will by claiming that he is *like* a person in a coma or a delerium. He is unable properly to respond to or comprehend a request for consent. Thus, the protests of such a person against being thrust into the sick role are ignored.

It is important to note the nature of this rhetorical device. The psychiatrist does not assert that mentally ill persons are comatose or delerious; he asserts that they *should be treated as if they are*, which is to say they should be treated without their consent and their protests should be viewed as the irresponsible babblings of men who are "out of their minds." This strategy makes it appear as if the psychiatrist's actions are justified by the patient's condition. Actually, the patient's "psychiatric condition," as incapable of giving consent, is *created* by the psychiatrist's unwillingness to require consent before "treatment." To borrow a metaphor from Ralph Ellison, who knew that he was invisible only because people refused to see him, the mental patient cannot give consent only because the psychiatrist refuses to request it or to honor the patient's protests about being treated against his will.[20] By transferring a medical situation into the context of psychiatry, the psychiatrist is able to justify involuntary hospitalization and treatment by saying that his patients are no more capable of giving consent than are persons who are unconscious or delerious.

Another device used by psychiatrists to justify involuntary hospitalization and treatment is stretching the definition of childhood. Children may be medically treated against their will provided that permission is granted by their parents or a court. Psychiatrists often justify the treatment of an adult without his consent by claiming that, as the result of mental illness, he has regressed to, or become fixated at the emotional level of a child. The statement that an adult is an emotional child may thus be used to deprive him of his rights as an adult and coercively to modify his behavior. However, the age at which an individual acquires his rights is determined by state law and not by psychiatric fiat. The law does not require that an individual emotionally reach the legal age, merely that he chronologically reach it. This psychiatric device ignores the legal definition of adulthood and the civil rights of adults. It is made socially palatable by defining certain adults as childlike and then following the acceptable medical practice of treating "children" against their will.

In medicine, the concepts of health and disease represent positive and negative ideals, rather than objective, scientifically discovered states. Medical interventions are organized social efforts to realize these ideals. This is also true in psychiatry. However, there are important differences between medicine and psychiatry.

The most important difference is that in medicine, the concepts of health and disease refer to bodily states. In psychiatry they refer to social conduct. Bodily states are classified as medical diseases on the basis of the desire to intervene in processes that are associated with pain, physical disability, and death. Social conduct is classified as mental diseases on the basis of the desire to intervene in the life of an individual who is personally distressed, or who distresses others by his behavior.

The psychiatric concepts of mental health and illness have an ethical basis as do physical health and illness in medicine. Since the psychiatric use of these terms refers to behavior, it is clear that the meaning of "mental illness" is "undesirable behavior." The meaning of "mental health" is "desirable behavior." The distinction between mental health and mental illness therefore, is a paralegal, cryptomoral distinction between desirable and undesirable behavior.

Because the term "mental illness" refers to social conduct, it may be used to label any behavior as undesirable and the person exhibiting such behavior as in need of corrective action. Similarly, any behavior deemed desirable may be designated as "health." The interventions for transforming the undesirable to the desirable, "disease" to "health," may be described as "psychiatric technology." The rhetoric of health and disease is thus flexible enough to encompass all human activities. Psychiatric rhetoric may be used to justify social interventions in the name of the unimpeachable (and often unintelligable) authority of scientific (or medical) technology, rather than in the name of explicit social values and interests.

The medical disguise of psychiatry makes it easy to smuggle in a number of social functions under the guise of medical treatment. In the guise of a physician, the psychiatrist may function as a policeman, a warden, a parent, a minister, an educator, a personnel manager, and a scientific expert on human behavior. Each of these activities is based on inexplicit social values and social purposes, which must be understood in the context of our social rather than our medical institutions.

CHAPTER FOUR

━━━━━━━━━━━━━━━━━━━━━

The Social Matrix of Psychiatry

━━━━━

> I am suggesting that the nature of the patient's nature is redefined so that, in effect if not by intention, the patient becomes the kind of object upon which a psychiatric service can be performed.
>
> —ERVING GOFFMAN[1]

━━━━━

Psychiatry is more influenced by social and ethical factors than is medicine. The diagnosis of medical illness is based on the evaluation of an individual's body in the light of his desire to live a long life free from pain and disability. The diagnosis of mental illness is based on the evaluation of an individual's behavior in the light of society's desire that its members conform to accepted norms of conduct. Thus, in the case of psychiatric "pathology," to quote Goffman: ". . . decisions concerning it tend to be political, in the sense of expressing the social interest of some particular faction or person rather than interests that can be said to be above the concerns of any particular groupings, as in the case of physical pathology."[2]

The social matrix of psychiatry is exceedingly complex. The

use of the concept of mental illness depends on complicated historical, sociological, economic, ethical, and political factors. By leading us to believe that mental illness is similar to physical illness and that psychiatry is similar to medicine, the medical model helps to obscure the relationship of psychiatry to these complex factors. As a result, historians have interpreted psychiatry primarily in the context of the history of medicine. The medical model has influenced them to examine certain past *social* events as if they were actually early, unenlightened, psychiatric practices.[3] Thus, medical historians of psychiatry have unwittingly served to disguise the social functions of psychiatry in the mask of medicine.

Since history is written in the context of some contemporary perspective or problem,[4] the history of psychiatry will be written differently if it is viewed from a social rather than from a medical perspective. If early psychiatric practices were understood in the context of critical and complex changes in the character of Western civilization, it would be easier to understand the social functions of contemporary psychiatry and the ideological functions of the medical model.

A SOCIAL AND HISTORICAL PERSPECTIVE
ON CONTEMPORARY PSYCHIATRY

In the earliest times there was the intimate group affiliation variously described as "The Little Community," "The Folk Society,"[5] "The Gemeinschaft,"[6] "The Status Society,"[7] "The Relationship of Mechanical Solidarity,"[8] and "The Primitive Society."[9]

This ancient social pattern has, with time and social change, been transformed into the modern mass society that, by contrast, has been labelled the Secular Society, the Urban Society, the Gesellschaft, the Contract Society, and the Relationship of Organic Solidarity.[10] The transition from ancient to modern social arrangements is associated with a number of now familiar developments: secularization, demythologization, bureaucratization, specialization, industrialization, urbanization, and alienation. Each of these developments constitutes a complex subject in itself, too complex to be detailed here. It is enough to emphasize that the history of psychiatry must be traced through the interstices of these developments.

Perhaps the most important outcome of these historical changes is the emergence of the individual and the collective (particularly the state) as the primary social units. This is of the utmost importance, for it accounts for contradictions and tensions in modern society that cannot be understood otherwise.

From the point of view of the individual, both gains and losses result from the transition from communal to modern forms of social life. On the one hand, the individual has gained his liberty from the oppressive bonds of traditional authority and obligation and has won an increasing mastery over nature. On the other hand, he has lost a secure social bond and feels the terror of his new cultural nakedness, cosmic loneliness, and alienation. In response to the evils associated with the loss of community, human energies and visions have mobilized both quiet and turbulent social movements in search of ". . . a millenial sense of participation in heavenly power on earth."[11] These utopian movements have generally been of two contradictory types—those that sponsor the transcendent individual and those that sponsor a new, collective moral order. In the course of the search for a better future the values of individual freedom and responsibility have come into morbid conflict with the values of the collective regulation of social and economic life.

These basic themes are fundamental to the development of psychiatry as a social institution. In particular, two aspects of these historical shifts are directly relevant to the emergence of modern psychiatry—the transformation in the character of social power and mechanisms of social control and the erosion of the traditional structures for guiding and evaluating human conduct. These changes are, of course, intimately and intricately interwoven with each other and, indeed, with the entire fabric of our culture.

Psychiatry and the Transformation of Social Power

The unity and harmony of primitive life is its most striking contrast to modern societies. The religious, economic, political, and social aspects of life were blended into a single fabric in which the individual participated with all the dimensions of his being. Primitive unity was not a logical coherence but an aesthetic and dramatic whole. It was not abstract but personal. Lived participation in the relatedness of all things was deeply ingrained and celebrated in all dimensions of life.

In primitive societies human relationships took precedence over those with property. The individual's relationship to the group was mediated by the primary associated structures—the family, the clan, and the small settlement. Authority and social control were exercised in face-to-face encounters with elders, kin, chiefs, shamans, and priests. Regulation of conduct was rooted in kinship and custom, in status and obligation, and in ethics and etiquette. Although punishment was often cruel and arbitrary, it was intimate and personal as in the contemporary family.[12]

The agricultural revolution initiated a complicated chain of events that profoundly altered the primitive social world.[13] Increased food supply led gradually to an increase in population; relief from food-gathering obligations; the specialization of skills, labor, and social functions; a money economy; and class stratification based on occupation and property ownership.[14] With an increase in travel, trade, and social mobility, divergent traditions mixed with and diluted one another and specialized governmental structures developed to regulate and conduct trade, to levy taxes, to perform public works, and to raise armies for defense and conquest. The result was the weakening of family and kinship ties, the emergence of the disaffiliated individual, and the transfer of social authority to the state. In contrast to the clan and community, the state is a large, impersonal, bureaucratically organized collectivity.

The dissolution of the primary associative bonds and the dilution and weakening of traditional values, standards and myths contributed to the progressive social unmooring and cultural defrocking of the individual. Only in this nakedness, in the circumstances of an experienced loss of a coherent cultural environment (alienation) could man discover that vital part of his nature created by and in culture. Yet, the conditions of this self-discovery are also the conditions in which the modern individual experiences moral uncertainty, confusion of identity, and existential anxiety.[15] Having been separated from a cultural form that animated both nature and himself, man developed a troubled sense that life was ebbing from nature[16] and from God.[17]

At the same time, the emergence of the individual as a social unit gave rise to a spirit of humanism and individual freedom. The political structure delegated with the task of preserving this spirit was constitutional government based on the principles of contract and Rule of Law. In one sense, government by Rule of Law is anarchic in that it serves as a restraint on the arbitrary use of power by the state. The centralization of authority and power in the state and the simultaneous valuation of individual freedom, which requires a restraint on the use of that power, combined to create a deep tension in Western civilization that has been a major factor in the development of modern psychiatry.

In spite of the transfer of civil authority to the state and the transcription of moral standards into law, many elements of traditional morality persist not codified in law. Guidelines for conduct in modern societies are provided both by contract (law) and by traditional forms of obligation (morals), some of which are explicit and others not. Formerly, guidelines for conduct were enforced by family, clan, and community authority. Now many guidelines are unenforceable because the family structure is weakened and because the state must avoid framing laws so strict that they violate our sense of individual freedom.

While this society values Rule of Law and the individual freedoms it safeguards, it is disturbed by and demands control of behavior that is not illegal but violates certain traditional standards of social deportment. Yet with the decline of those social structures which formerly enforced those standards, this society lacks effective legitimate machinery for this control.

These circumstances required a new social institution that, under the auspices of an acceptable modern authority, could inconspicuously and with justification supplement the social control provided by law without violating publicly avowed ideals of individual freedom. Psychiatry is perfectly suited for this task.

By adopting the medical model, psychiatry can offer the credentials of the biophysical sciences. It may thus trade on the prestige and influence of modern science, which is replacing the authority of religious belief, myth, and dogma as the source of "certainty" and "truth." By using the crypto-ethical rhetoric of health and disease, psychiatrists have codified social standards of conduct in scientific-sounding language. Behavior that violates a social sense of propriety, safety, and stability may be labelled as mentally ill; behavior that is proper, safe, and productive may be labelled as mentally healthy. The social utility of the medical model in psychiatry is thus that psychiatric activities are classified as scientific and medical, rather than as social and ethical. This, in turn, permits the substitution of scientific (or medical) authority for social authority. It permits social authority to mask itself with scientific credentials and scientific credibility.

As "experts" in the modern "science" of human engineering, psychiatrists enforce standards of conduct by two methods. First, they may deface and stigmatize persons who violate these standards by labelling such persons as mentally ill. In spite of attempts to "educate" the public to the contrary, the label of mental illness is unlike that of medical illness in that mental illness carries the implication of social deviance. It implies, also, that the individual to whom it is ascribed is not responsible for his actions. There is no more devastating form of social defacement than to treat a man's actions as the irrelevant utterings and gestures of a madman.

Second, psychiatrists may enforce social standards by involuntary commitment. Under the guise of providing medical diagnostic and treatment services for the mentally ill, psychiatrists may detain, punish, and "correct" persons who, while they may have violated no law, have nevertheless transgressed certain rules of social demeanor. Involuntary mental hospitalization thus affords a greater degree of social control and protection for the community than is provided by laws that must avoid being so strict that they violate the principle of individual freedom.

In this function, psychiatrists join with and serve as the agents of the state. This partnership is achieved by mental health laws that, in a vague and undefined manner, legitimize the detention and confinement of persons who are suspected of being "mentally ill" and by the state's establishing, funding, and administering a vast network of psychiatric "hospitals." The power of the psychiatrist to stigmatize individuals and to confine them in mental hospitals is well known and hangs like Damocles' Sword over anyone who is the object of his professional attention.

Psychiatry and the Erosion of
Traditional Guidelines of Conduct

An important function of culture is to guide and evaluate human conduct. This is accomplished by a dramatical, social design that gives action meaning and that regulates conduct by means of directive and avoidance systems and hierarchies of value. Systems of social authority inculcate obligations, enforce standards, and guide and correct behavior.[18] Changes in the institutional forms of social authority will inevitably have an impact on the behavior of the individuals who are the ultimate target of its influence. The impact of the larger cultural design on individual behavior, however, is far more crucial, and transformations of this design will penetrate to the deepest core of the human character.

Three related aspects of cultural design are particularly important for individual behavior: *cultural coherence*—the harmonious relationship of the various elements of a culture; *cultural simplicity*—the nonspecialization and nondifferentiation of a culture that permits the individual to have personal acquaintance with its various dimensions; and *personal freedom*—the expanded range of permissable alternatives in personal conduct.

Social conduct will be less problematical and uncertain for the individual the more coherent and simple the cultural design and the more authoritarian the social structure. Conversely, the burdens of choice-making will increase for the individual as the cultural design becomes more incoherent and contradictory, as the culture becomes more complex and differentiated, and as the idea of personal freedom becomes a social reality.

Among primitives, the socialization process involved the intimate encounter of children with virtually all of the dimensions of a well-defined, well-bounded, relatively undifferentiated cultural territory. In such small groups, where individuals were able to participate so widely in social activities, young people could gain a personal knowledge of almost all adult social roles.[19] The rules of social conduct were clearly set forth by the obligations of status and custom. The social environment was relatively stable, predictable, and undisturbed by cross-cultural influences. Significant social choices were guided by precedent, group opinion, and the authority of elders, shamans, and chiefs. The daily round of life was a comparatively harmonious integration of the economic, social, political, and religious elements of existence. It was anchored in moral certainty and a coherent world view, and it was ratified in myth and ceremony.

With the decline of community and the development of

the modern, industrial society the complexity, incoherence, and permissiveness of the social environment have increased immeasurably.[20] As a result, the individual has experienced a diminishing sense of familiarity and mastery of his cultural territory and he has experienced an increasing sense of estrangement from the sources of social power, values, norms, from nature, from God, from other men, and from himself.[21]

Thus, modern life has increased the difficulties and hazards of growing up. The weakening of the traditional primary group—the extended family and clan—has also weakened the major mechanism for socializing and educating the young. This burden is now largely assumed by the nuclear family—a poorly socially integrated unit—and by the school—a highly structured, impersonal bureaucracy.

The rapidity of social change creates an increasing incompatibility between patterns of socialization and the complex requirements of adult life. This results not only in discontinuities and conflicts between the generations, but also in the near obsolescence of socialization as soon as it is completed.[22] Moreover, the family and school function as authoritarians to whose values the child is obliged to conform (or rebel). Consequently, the adult is subject to deep psychological conflicts. On the one hand he feels a sense of obligation to conform his behavior to familial and school standards; on the other hand, he feels justified by the spirit of freedom and changing social values to make new and creative choices. Although the individual is socially emancipated from ancestral and even familial authority, his newly won freedoms are associated with an increase in psychological conflicts and problems of choice-making. The personal freedom of others has diminished the stability and predictability of his social environment.

Under these circumstances, the confusions and casualties of social life were bound to increase, and new methods for dealing with these problems had to be developed. One method was the transformation of the relationship between

God and man. In primitive societies, the spirits presided primarily over nature. Their help was often sought in matters of hunting, agriculture, medicine, and war, but less frequently in relations between men.[23] In civil societies, on the other hand, the reverse is true. The power and authority of God is not relevant to our understanding of or interventions in the physical universe. However, He is deeply involved in relations between men.[24]

With the increasing secularization of Western culture, religious methods for guiding and evaluating conduct have lost much of their influence. Psychiatry has taken up the slack. By means of psychotherapy, the modern, "scientific" method of spiritual direction, psychiatrists may provide supplemental socialization and educational experiences to individuals who are judged to be unprepared (or unwilling) to meet the complicated opportunities and obligations of modern life.[25] Thus, psychiatry may be construed as a secular, pseudo-scientific priesthood, which by codifying rules for evaluating and guiding conduct as principles of mental hygiene, provides a secular ethic for modern man, who, having lost the guidelines of traditional social authority, eagerly grasps for substitutes from the modern authority of science.

Psychiatry has assumed, in a medical disguise, three historical social functions. First, it has assumed a part of the function of controlling human behavior by the exercise of social power. This power is provided by an alliance with Science and the State—the one being the prevalent social "mythology," the other the prime repository of social power. Second, psychiatry has assumed a large portion of the function of guiding and evaluating human conduct. For this purpose, contemporary psychiatrists employ both "primitive" and modern methods—charismatic influence, shame, defacement, stigmatization, conditioning (influencing behavior with rewards and punishments), the inculcation of conscience, casuistry, drugs, shock therapy and confinement. Third, with psychonalysis, psychiatry assumes the relatively new function of assisting the individual to achieve a transcendence of conscience and an increased self-mastery over the problems of living in the modern world.

To see the influence of social, political, and economic factors on the development of psychiatry and the use of the medical model, three important phases of the history of psychiatry—primitive psychiatry, hospital psychiatry, and psychoanalysis and psychotherapy—will be briefly reinterpreted.

A BRIEF HISTORY OF PSYCHIATRY

Primitive Psychiatry

To view the primitive psychiatrist or shaman primarily as a medicine man who attempted to cure disease by magical means is a mistake. Robert Lowie writes of the shaman:

> To all intents and purposes, the shamanistic leader of the secret organization was the most eminent person in the community. He regulated the ceremonial life of his people, adjusted disputes, insured a good corn crop, warded off disease and by his magical powers inflicted condign punishment on the enemy: indeed, he himself often led war parties in person. Over and above all these things, he was the authority on tribal mythology and lore, and it was his duty to instruct the people on these lofty topics.[26]

The prominence of the shaman was not based solely on his special knowledge about disease and his skills in curing it. His special status was due primarily to his possession of socially useful power. He was believed to be in contact with the spirits and forces of the universe, to be able to enlist their aid, and to influence them.

The kind of social power exercised by the primitive psychiatrist was related to the structure of his society. Primitive modes of dealing with deviance, including mental illness, have been characterized by Levi-Strauss as "cannibalistic."

By this he means that the social response to persons engaging in deviant, threatening, or incomprehensible behavior was most often to attempt to bring them more fully into the "body" of the group. Primitive societies, therefore, had no mental hospitals. Some societies did have sick huts, but where they did exist, they were not places of exile but rather an integral part of the community. Mental hospitals develop only where the community and family begin to disintegrate and where methods of controlling deviance become "anthropoemic" (from the Greek: emein—to vomit.) By this term, Levi-Strauss refers to modern (alienating) methods for the treatment of the mentally ill in which we: ". . . expel these formidable beings from the body public by isolating them for a time, or forever, denying them all contact with humanity, in establishments devised for that express purpose."[27]

At one level, we may say that primitive methods for bringing the mentally ill person back into the group involve the use of magic and faith. Paul Radin,[28] however, described the goal of primitive magic as "the coercion of the world." At a deeper level, magic and faith may be construed as subtle devices of intimidation and coercion. They coerce people as well as Nature and Gods.

In treating physical disease, the shaman's interventions may have an instrumental effect on the disease process, for instance by draining an abscess.[29] In such cases, modern man would explain the cure with theories of medical science, although the primitive might attempt to explain it in magical terms. In the absence of a medical (physical) explanation of the shaman's success, for instance in treating "mental illness," the effect on the patient must be explained in terms of the shaman's influence over him.[30] This influence is based largely on the shaman's powers and the patient's "illness" being conceptualized the same way by both persons according to the same "assumptive system."[31] The faith of the participants in this assumptive system is an important instrument of social control! It obliges an individual to do what he can to bring about what he believes should occur.

Faith is important in treating "mental illness" because (as far as we know) no physicochemical processes stand in the way of "cure." All that is required is for the individual to alter his behavior. The shaman's social status and the faith of the tribe in his legitimacy exert pressure on the patient to alter his behavior in the desired direction. The patient who believes in the magic of the shaman is provided with a powerful motive for recovery, for if he fails to recover he runs the risk of being perceived as "unforgiven" by the Gods, as having committed an unpardonable sin. This view has something in common with the modern notion of "incurable" mental illness. Each concept, the "unforgiven" and the "incurable," serves to protect the reputation of the shaman's and the psychiatrist's efficacy.

Treatment of the mentally ill in primitive societies may involve the group as well as the shaman. Clan rituals, feasts, and celebrations may be employed to effect a cure.[32] For instance, the Shona of Rhodesia make the mentally ill person the guest of honor at a feast. He receives food, drink, and gifts for days on end, while his family and friends persuade and cajole him until, exhausted and ashamed, he abandons his deviant beliefs and actions. These methods are thinly disguised forms of social coercion and differ only slightly from modern techniques of brainwashing.

The shaman is the historical predecessor of the modern psychiatrist not because he possessed early and unsophisticated psychiatric knowledge and techniques, but because the categories with which primitive religion dealt have become differentiated into a number of modern social functions, one group of which is exercised by the modern psychiatrist.[33] Among these functions are social control, moral guidance, and formulating mythologies.

The primitive predecessors of the contemporary psychiatrist were men of considerable social power. The modern psychiatrist differs from the shaman not because he has abandoned social power for medical science, but because he has disguised his power with the rhetoric of medicine and science instead of magic and religion. In this sense, historical interpretations of the shaman that emphasize his healing functions instead of his social influence and power are misleading. They tend to reinforce current use of the medical model for understanding the modern psychiatrist instead of lending evidence that the psychiatrist has always functioned as an agent of social intervention.

Hospital Psychiatry

Mental hospitals are the products of civilization. They made their appearance in history along with the city. There were at least three main effects of the transformation from primitive to modern society. First, it resulted in the emergence of the individual as a new social unit. As the individual was wrested from the moorings of community, his vulnerability to social, economic, and psychological disasters increased. At the same time, he was placed in the new milieu of a stratified society where class conflict, exploitation, and collective power increased his jeopardy.

Second, the influence of community, clan, and family declined. As these units lost their influence, they became less able to perform their previous functions, which included the control and regulation of behavior and the care of those who could not or did not work.

Third, Church and State gradually assumed many of the functions of the family and community. Among these were the enforcement of standards of conduct, the care of poor and ill persons, and the punishment and control of deviance.[34] The mental hospital developed in this social context.

To consider early temples of healing to be the predecessors of the modern mental hospital is erroneous. Medical and mental hospitals have different social origins. Early medical hospitals were primarily for *voluntary* patients, including the poor. Until the end of the Middle Ages, there were few

special provisions for the mentally ill. The mental hospital
began as an institution of *involuntary* confinement for lower
class persons.

It is true that during the Middle Ages, occasional religious
orders provided food and asylum for the homeless and inept.
For the most part, however, as George Henry writes:

> Those who were shunned by their fellow beings wan-
> dered about in lonely places at night and remained in
> hiding during the day. Some of the more excited and
> violent were flogged and confined with chains, occa-
> sionally without human contact except at such times
> as food might be thrown to them. Those who were
> mild mannered were permitted to wander about freely,
> the subjects of ridicule, pity, or, at times, even venera-
> tion.[35]

The majority of persons of that day who, in retrospect we
label as mentally ill, were ostracized, bothersome, ill-man-
nered wanderers. Even while scorning this Medieval attitude
toward the "mentally ill," Henry betrays the difference between them and the physically ill. He states: "When it
became *necessary to deal with* the mentally sick, they were
usually confined in prisons, in buildings which were no longer
considered suitable as monasteries, or in former pesthouses."[36]
(Italics added.) The physically ill required treatment; but the
"mentally ill" were "necessary to deal with." This illustrates
that the "treatment of the mentally ill" began and continues
in the context of social control.

The legions of the poor, homeless and unemployed were
multiplied by the social dislocations of centuries—by war,
famine, plague, political and economic oppression, and exploitation. The distance widened between the rich and powerful classes and the poor and powerless classes. By one estimate,
there were more than 30,000 beggars in Paris out of a population of less than 100,000 at the end of the sixteenth century.[37]
By 1791, there were 118,000 indigents out of a population of
650,000.[38] To the bourgeoisie, beggars were offensive con-

taminants of the city who refused to be inconspicuous, to overcome their sloth, or to consign themselves voluntarily to flames as so much human refuse. They were demanding children who, in effect, levied taxes with their pleas for alms while they lived in idleness and a state of moral libertinism.

The power of the State was used to eliminate these "annoyances" whose causes led, one century later, to the French Revolution.[39] Mental hospitals developed in the context of an undisguised war on the poor, the homeless, the unemployed, and the morally deviant. This war was waged primarily by the State through punishment, confinement, and exile. The predecessors of the modern mental hospital were the almshouse, the leprosarium, the prison, and the *Hôpital General*.

Michel Foucault gives the year of 1656 as the landmark of this war.[40] By the end of the Crusades there were approximately 1900 leprosariums in Europe. Leprosy had virtually disappeared from Europe by the end of the Middle Ages, and these facilities were available as institutions of confinement. In 1656 a decree established the *Hôpital General* in Paris from a variety of existing Parisian institutions, including the famous hospitals La Salpetriere and Bicetre.

The inmates of the *Hôpital* were largely the poor people of Paris who either admitted themselves voluntarily or were committted by Royal or judicial decree. Within a few months of its establishment, Foucault writes, one of every hundred citizens of Paris were inmates of the *Hôpital General*. In 1657, after a long series of suppressive laws, begging was prohibited in Paris; those who were caught by the "archers of the *Hôpital*" were either whipped, branded, exiled, killed, or confined.[41] In 1676, by Royal decree, a *Hôpital General* was established in every sizable city in France. This process was much the same across the European continent.

Although a physician was appointed to visit each of the houses of the *Hôpital* twice a week, there was no pretense that the inmates were confined for medical treatment. Foucault states:

> From the very start, one thing is clear: the *Hôpital General* is not a medical establishment. It is rather a sort of a semijudicial structure, an administrative entity which, along with the already constituted powers, and outside of the courts, decides, judges, and executes. "The directors having for these purposes stakes, irons, prisons, and dungeons in the said *Hôpital General* . . ." A quasi-absolute sovereignty, jurisdiction without appeal, a writ of execution against which nothing can prevail—the *Hôpital General* is a strange power that the King establishes between the police and the courts, at the limits of the law: a third order of repression. *The insane whom Pinel would find at Bicetre and at La Salpetriere belonged to this world.*[42]

The function of these institutions was clearly stated in ordinary language, unencumbered by mental health rhetoric. The explicit purpose of the act that established the Hôpital General was to "prevent mendicancy and idleness as the source of all disorders."[43] An act of 1575, in England, defined the new asylums as for the purpose of "the punishment of the vagabonds and the relief of the poor."[44]

In addition to serving as concentration camps for the poor, these infamous houses performed other economic, social, political, and moral functions. They dealt with the problem of unemployment, and therefore with the riots associated with it, by removing the obnoxious poor from the labor force. In periods of higher employment, they served as cheap sources of forced labor for institutions that manufactured the special products of their locale. The inmates also often provided a cheap source of labor for private enterpreneurs who rented them from the state. The houses also served to punish and reform immoral and antisocial persons. This was accomplished by means of physical and mental torture and by means of "work therapy" in accordance with the Protestant belief that work was both penance and redemption.[45]

Another function of confinement in the *Hôpital* consisted of the Orwellian practice of creating nonpersons. An individual who was committed to an asylum was thereby stigmatized and defaced; he was made into a nonperson who, indeed, might never be seen or heard from again. The reasons for his behavior were rendered insignificant and irrelevant. If his actions were (or could be construed as) social protests, as cries against injustice, or as pleas for the redress of grievances, the evils to which they referred need not be confronted. Instead, the motives for his actions and the meaning of his complaints could be interpreted as the wild fantasies of the insane and hidden from public view. Thus, social scandals could be avoided and conduct that might be socially provocative could be defined as nonconduct.[46]

Foucault states:

> Hence, the *Hôpital* does not have the appearance of a mere refuge for those whom age, infirmity, or sickness keep from working; it will have not only the aspect of a forced labor camp, but also that of a moral institution responsible for punishing, for correcting a certain moral "abeyance" which does not merit the tribunal of men, but cannot be corrected by the severity of penance alone.[47]

Until the French Revolution, the state had unlimited power to confine and punish those who offended the bourgeois and Royal sense of propriety and morality. With the Revolution, however, the political climate changed. A law of 1790 suppressed the *lettres de cachet* and the *ordres arbitraires*. The new spirit of "Liberty, Equality, Fraternity" permeated even the dungeons of the *Hôpital General*, culminating in 1793 in the famous reforms of Philippe Pinel in the Bicetre. At that point, it became necessary to redefine formally, the nature of the lunatic so that the state could continue to confine and punish him. The medical model was conveniently ready and waiting to be put to this use.

The view that "mentally ill" persons were possessed by demons and the view that they were ill were both useful as justifications for the involuntary confinement of threatening and undesirable persons. However, the demonological model was under challenge; the medical model had the advantage of being more in harmony with the scientific and intellectual climate of the day. As an ideology, it was well suited to compensate for the new mandate for humane reform by disguising and justifying the continued use of state power to confine the poor and the morally wayward. Also, since physicians were the main professional group to come into intimate contact with the inmates of asylums, the medical model prevailed as the preferred system for explaining and classifying the behavior of "lunatics."

Following the French Revolution, the practice of harassing and persecuting the poor was reformulated as a policy of community responsibility to establish state social welfare programs for them. The asylum became a mental hospital as a result of the same reformulation. Instead of being defined as houses of confinement in which inmates were removed from society, punished, reformed, and pressed into labor, mental institutions were redefined as hospitals to provide care and treatment for the mentally ill. This change consisted of social and rhetorical reforms rather than innovations in medical treatment or alterations of the basic social dynamics and social functions of the asylum.[48] Pinel and his fellow psychiatric "revolutionaries," as is the mental hospital administrator of today, were jailers who ruled with absolute authority over persons who had been deprived of their liberty against their will and without trial or due process.

In the rush to congratulate psychiatrists as humane reformers, the role of Philippe Pinel has not been given a balanced examination. For instance, Zilboorg and Henry,[49] in their *History of Medical Psychology*, do not mention Pinel's reference to the chief manager of the hospital, the Bicetre, to which Pinel was appointed as chief physician. The impression is given that Pinel was responsible for the humane reforms that took place at this institution. However, Pinel himself describes his anonymous superior as ". . . a kind and affectionate parent" who ". . . . never lost sight of the principles of a most genuine philanthropy."[50] One infers from Pinel's account that the manager was not a physician. Why was this man not given at least partial credit for the humane reforms at the Bicetre? Is it possible that Dr. Pinel and not his unnamed, nonmedical superior, was remembered as the genuine humanitarian to certify that the reforms were medical rather than social in nature?

Zilboorg and Henry and other psychiatric historians also do not mention Pinel's fondness for coercion. For instance, Pinel gives the history of a law student who, he believes, might have been saved from suicide if he had been committed to an asylum in which he would be ". . . subject to the management of a governor, in every respect qualified to exercise over him an irresistible control."[51] Elsewhere in his *Treatise*, Pinel vigorously praises "The estimable effects of coercion . . ."[52] He states: "To render the effects of fear solid and durable, its influence ought to be associated with that of a profound regard. For that purpose, plots must either be avoided or so well managed to be the result of necessity, reluctantly resorted to and commensurate with the violence or petulance which it is intended to correct."[53] These words have a contemporary relevance for both the expert in techniques of brainwashing and in coercive "psychotherapy." It is clear from his writings that, contrary to the favorable publicity that he has received, Pinel was opposed only to coercion that was not redeemed by the psychiatrist's good intentions. In the use of this new rhetoric to justify coercion, Pinel was indeed the revolutionary predecessor of the modern hospital psychiatrist.

The social changes of the French Revolution did not alter the continued public demand for confinement and control of persons who exhibited bizarre, unconventional, and dangerous breaches of social ethics and etiquette. The legal and moral reforms of the Revolution made it less justifiable and more difficult arbitrarily to deprive a person of his liberty without first accusing him of a crime and providing him with a trial.

The medical rhetoric simplified this task. According to this rhetoric, involuntary confinement in a mental hospital was redefined as benefitting the inmate instead of society. He was *defined* as ill and unaware of his need for medical help, or unreasonably uncooperative in seeking it. He was therefore hospitalized against his will so that he could receive the "necessary" psychiatric treatment. The same social function that was openly performed for a thousand years, namely the control and correction of deviant behavior by means of confinement, was now covertly continued under a new medical rubric that satisfied the demands of the day for humane reform.

The social dynamics of the asylum of three hundred years ago, which Foucault could see with such faultless vision, are visible today in the modern European and American mental hospital to those who do not wear the filtering lenses of the medical model. (See chapter eight for a special treatment of the American mental hospital.) Public mental hospitals continue as places of confinement for primarily the lower socioeconomic classes.[54] In countries where unemployment is high, such as the United States, the "mentally ill" are committed to spend idle time watching television or weaving baskets and performing chores defined as "occupational therapy." In countries where unemployment is low, such as the Soviet Union, the "mentally ill" are often consigned to forced labor camps.[55] That mental hospitals continue to function as institutions of moral reform has also been noticed by those who have not been misled by the medical rhetoric.[56] Finally, the use of psychiatric defacement to avoid public discussion of sensitive and potentially scandalous issues has not been abandoned.[57]

The chains are gone, the beatings are less frequent and more secretive, the locked doors have been opened in many institutions, and the interior decorations have been improved. However, mental hospitals are still used primarily to confine disruptive members of the lower classes. The chains are chemical and legal, the beatings are psychological, and the locks have been replaced by members of the mental health team who guard the open doors.[58] The rapid discharge rate, far from being an index of the "progress" of medical psychiatry, is evidence of an increased efficiency in influencing and controlling thought and behavior.

Images of insanity have also changed. They have become secular and "scientific." The genetic taint has been transformed into a subtle, sophisticated (and as yet unidentified) metabolic defect; the source of evil has changed from demons and spirits to traumas of childhood and society. The obnoxious, immoral, and threatening act is viewed as the symptom of an insidious disease. The hospital psychiatrist, instead of being viewed as a jailer, warden, and moral reformer, is viewed as a humane physician who is intent on curing his ill patient. However, the social and historical nucleus of mental institutions, from the *Hôpital General* to the modern community mental health center, endures. They are instruments of the state employed for the involuntary confinement of persons who have offended the public sense of behavioral propriety.

Psychoanalysis and Psychotherapy

Before psychoanalysis, most psychiatrists worked in hospitals, many of them as government employees. They functioned as agents of families and communities, dealing with patients who were, for the most part, involuntary wards. The reverse was true in medicine, which most physicians practiced privately for a fee and as the agents of their voluntary patients.[59] Sigmund Freud, after a brilliant but frustrated beginning as a neuroanatomist and neurophysiologist, abandoned his career in scientific research for the private practice of medicine and neurology.[60] As a result, psychoanalysis developed in the social context of private medical practice. As did his medical colleagues, Freud worked for a fee and served only his private patients, who were free to terminate his services when they pleased. Unlike the hospital psychiatrist, Freud did not practice coercion or confinement and thus did not require the medical model to justify these actions. Why then, did he persist in using the medical model?

One reason was that the theories of biology and medicine were the most basic part of Freud's intellectual equipment. To understand how difficult it would have been for Freud to abandon the most successful theoretical model of his day in favor of a poorly articulated and less prestigious sociopsychological framework, one must appreciate the impact of his long years of training in physiology and medicine, as well as his strong ambition to make important contributions to science.

Very early in his career Freud recognized the differences between physical and mental illness. In describing the differences between organic paralysis and hysterical paralysis Freud stated:

> Again, every clinical detail of a representation [organic] paralysis finds its explanation in some detail of cerebral anatomy and, vice versa, we can deduce the structure of the brain from the clinical characteristics of the paralysis. We believe that a perfect parallel exists between these two series of facts.[61]

And:

> I maintain on the contrary that the lesions in hysterical paralysis must be entirely independent of the anatomy of the nervous system.[62]

To disguise these crucial differences between medical and mental illness and to continue to use the medical model to explain hysterical symptoms, Freud postulated a "functional lesion" that consisted in the absence of the *idea* of the paralyzed part in consciousness.[63] Thus began the problem of the "mysterious leap from the mind to the body" over which psychiatrists still puzzle.[64]

It is true, as Robert Holt suggests, that "many of the most

puzzling and seemingly arbitrary turns of psychoanalytic theory are either hidden biological assumptions or result directly from such assumptions . . . When Freud replaced the explicitly physicalistic model of the Project with a psychological one he did so only partially and incompletely."[65] There is evidence, however, that Freud himself was troubled and ambivalent about the incongruities between his clinical data and his use of the medical model to explain them. In the case of Miss Elizabeth v. R., Freud wrote:

> I have not always been a psychotherapist, but like other neuro-pathologists I was educated to methods of focal diagnosis and electrical prognosis, so that even I myself am struck by the fact that the case histories which I am writing read like novels, and as it were, dispense with the serious features of the scientific character. Yet I must console myself with the fact that the nature of the subject is apparently more responsible for this issue than my own predilection.[66]

If, however, Freud realized that "the nature of the subject" did not lend itself to being described according to his predilections, in the language of the biological sciences, why did he not redefine his subject matter as nonmedical? Why did he not fully develop the implication of this observation that his case histories read like novels rather than like medical texts: that the phenomena of "mental illness" belonged in the context of human behavior rather than in the context of bodily disease?[67]

Freud's preference for the medical model cannot be attributed solely to his early training in the physical sciences. Early in his life he was also interested in politics and expressed a desire to study law.[68] Later, his readings of Darwin and Goethe influenced him to study medicine.[69] Freud retained his interest in philosophy, history and social affairs; in fact, very early in his career, he prepared a philosophical primer, entitled A Philosophical ABC, to acquaint his wife with his intellectual temperament.[70] In 1910, Freud expressed a wish to retire from medical practice and devote himself to the study of human nature and cultural problems. In 1927, he confessed:

> After forty-one years of medical activity my self-knowledge tells me that I have never really been a doctor in the proper sense . . . Nor did I ever play the "doctor game" . . . In my youth I felt an overpowering need to understand something of the riddles of the world in which we live and perhaps even to contribute something to their solution.[71]

Actually, Freud half abandoned the medical model by advocating the cause of lay analysis.[72] In a postscript to his discussion of this subject Freud stated:

> It will not have escaped my readers that in what I have said I have assumed as axiomatic something that is still violently disputed . . . I have assumed . . . that psychoanalysis is not a specialized branch of medicine. I cannot see how it is possible to dispute this. Psychoanalysis is a part of psychology; not of medical psychology in the old sense, not of the psychology of the morbid processes, but simply of psychology . . . The possibility of its application to medical purposes must not lead us astray. Electricity and radiology also have their medical application, but the science to which they both belong is nevertheless physics. Nor can the situation be affected by historical arguments . . . It is argued that psychoanalysis was after all discovered by a physician in the course of his efforts to assist his patients. But that is clearly neither here nor there.[73]

What were the "medical purposes" to which psychoanalysis was applied? If Freud's case histories read like novels, why did he not consider the troubles of their heroes and heroines as problems in living rather than as medical diseases? And surely, if Freud viewed his own psychoanalytic operations with the same literary eye, (as he did, on occasions) he would have seemed to be more like a priest, a critic, and an educator than like a physician. Why did Freud hedgingly define only his science and not also his practice as non-medical?

The principle reason Freud did not do this was economic! He needed patients to develop his science and to support his family and himself. "A physicist," he said, "does not require to have a patient in order to study the laws that govern X-rays. But the only subject matter of psychoanalysis is the mental process of human beings and it is only in human beings that it can be studied."[74] Freud raised this point to argue for training nonmedical persons in the science and techniques of psychoanalysis. However, *it applies equally well to himself.* Freud did not receive income from a university, nor did he have foundation grants that would have permitted him to pay subjects for scientific research. The only way in which Freud could obtain access to the subjects of his study and also earn a living was to avoid tampering with the popular definition of his patient's problems and his professional activities as medical.

In spite of his willingness to define psychoanalysis as a medical *practice,* the evidence suggests that Freud was more interested in science and money than in helping people. Freud's use of the medical model, which defined him as a physician and his patients as ill, did not serve a scientific or a medical purpose. It served the social and economic purposes of permitting him to have socially justifiable access to intimacy with persons who would pay him a fee to be the subject of his scientific inquiries.[75]

This socioeconomic explanation accounts for the present ambiguity about the use of the medical model in psychoanalysis and psychotherapy. In general, those for whom it is an economic advantage, define psychotherapy as a medical enterprise and they define their patients as mentally ill. Those for whom this would be a disadvantage define psychotherapy as nonmedical and they view their clients as suffering from problems in living. There are secondary advantages to the use of the medical model for the modern psychotherapist. Medical physicians and physical scientists are regarded with great esteem in our society. Without their medical mantle, psychotherapists would be grouped with social scientists, literary critics, welfare workers, and the ministry—on the whole a less prestigious group that commands a lower price for their services. Also, the claims of therapists might be deprived of "the serious stamp of science" and their social power and status, which is to a large degree derived from their status as scientific authorities, would be accordingly diminished.

What would be the historical significance of psychoanalysis and psychotherapy if they were not viewed in the context of medicine? Psychoanalytic theory and the contemporary mental hygiene doctrines have become the successors to the submerged religious myths with which the human drama was formerly represented and directed. They provide the modern lexicon for penetrating beyond the apparent and the obvious to the "deeper truths"—to the mysteries of being human. In fact, psychiatry has become more relevant to contemporary life than has religion. They have had reciprocal careers—psychiatry has waxed as religion has waned. Psychoanalytic and psychiatric theories have translated religious values into a universal, secular, value-free, scientific lexicon, and they have functionally replaced religious precepts for guiding and evaluating human conduct. Among increasing numbers of educated people, mental health slogans, aphorisms, and principles have become the guiding precepts for everyday activities. The concern is no longer with what is good for a man's soul, with what will insure his salvation, or with what will please God. Indeed, concern is decreasing as to whether or not a man has violated law, with whether or not proper legal procedures have governed our actions toward him, or with whether or not he has been accorded the dignity and responsibility of an adult in a free society. Instead, concern is for what is good for his mental health, for discovering his hidden mental illness, and for assuring that he will receive enough psychiatric treatment.

Sigmund Freud did not discover a new form of mental

illness. He discovered the troubled, disaffiliated modern individual in conflict. Sigmund Freud did not invent a new form of medical treatment. He invented a new social situation in which the troubled individual could become acquainted with the inexplicit and complex difficulties of growing up, with the intricacies of modern social life, and with new methods for guiding his conduct in an intelligent and self-controlled manner. The psychotherapist, in other words, is a modern successor to the shaman, the priest, the casuist, and the pastor.

Freud knew this well. He said "Indeed, the words, 'secular pastoral worker' might well serve as a general formula for describing the function which the analyst, whether he is a doctor or a layman, has to perform in relation to the public."[76]

THE PSEUDOLOGIC OF THE
EXPANSION OF PSYCHIATRIC NOSOLOGY

The history of psychiatry could well be written as the history of the expansion of psychiatric nosology. Each time psychiatrists have assumed a new social role they have invented a new mental illness to justify their new functions. The catalogue of psychiatric syndromes is thus the product of historical development rather than of logical refinement.

Classification is a sorting operation that depends on the purposes of the classifier as well as on the properties of the thing classified.[77] The basic element of this sorting process is that entities classified together must be similar in some respect. However, this is not a restrictive rule, since any two objects in the universe are similar to each other in some way. The similarity selected as the basis of classification, therefore, depends primarily on the purposes of the classifier. In "pure" scientific classification, that is, in sorting for the purpose of understanding, the classifier must attempt to divorce his purpose from any particular social context; his purpose must not serve any particular individual or group interests. This is obviously much easier to accomplish in the physical and biological sciences than in the social sciences. A classical example of pure scientific classification is the catalogue of the animal species in which *all* animals are categorized according to similarities of their bodily structure (rather than, for instance, according to their value to man as sources of food or material). Another example is the classification of the elements of which *all* of the simplest constituents of chemical reactions are categorized according to their unit weight (rather than according to their economic value.)

The major similarity of the "diseases" in the classification of mental illnesses is that they are all labels that have been applied, in their historical turn, only to persons who have become the objects of psychiatric attention and intervention. The purposes served by the classification of mental illnesses are therefore equivalent to the purposes served by psychiatrists. The class of mental illnesses is used to define certain persons as the kind of objects upon which psychiatric services may be performed (rather than to serve the purpose of understanding human behavior).

The first disorders classified as mental diseases were the organic brain syndromes. These disorders are distinguished by the fact that some pathological bodily process can be identified or presumed on good evidence to be the etiological factor. They are similar to other bodily diseases in this respect. Organic brain diseases differ from other medical diseases because they affect the brain and produce prominent psychological symptoms.

The second group to be classified as mental disorders was composed of the psychoses. The ancient Greeks and Romans recognized the manifestations of both organic brain diseases and psychoses, but most observers of that era attributed both disorders to pathological bodily processes, as do some contemporary psychiatrists. During the nineteenth and twentieth centuries, the psychoses were gradually "spun off" and differentiated from the organic brain diseases. Organic brain diseases have been associated with some distinctive bodily disease, while the psychoses are presumed either to be "functional," that is, caused by psychosocial factors, or to be caused by some yet unknown neurophysiological process.

The organic brain syndromes and the psychoses are both labels ascribed to persons who are considered to be (or potentially to be) severely socially incapacitated. During the era when psychiatry was practiced almost exclusively in institutions, subtypes of these two categories comprised the largest part of the nosology of mental illness. In describing the psychiatry of that era, Oskar Diethelm states:

> Little attention was paid to the many personality disorders which were not serious enough to cause the patient to enter a psychiatric hospital. It is consequently not surprising that psychosis and mental disease corresponded to "insanity" and "foli" and bore the connotation that the patient was committable.[78]

These two types of mental illness are still primarily associated with hospital psychiatry.

Although many neurotic symptoms had been described before Freud, the use of the psychoneuroses in the catalogue of psychiatric diseases was not popular until the advent of psychoanalysis. The category of psychoneuroses developed in the social context of the private practice of psychotherapy. Indeed, Freud's patients, for the most part, were not so socially disabled that they required hospitalization, or else they were wealthy and influential enough to avoid the public mental hospital.

It is significant that the first neurotics with whom Freud dealt were hysterics. Hysterics sometimes resemble persons with genuine neurological disease and are thus likely to come to the attention of a neurologist. Although Freud recognized the differences between conversion hysteria and organic neurological disorders, he did not consider the differences sufficient to distinguish conversion hysteria as a nonmedical phenomenon. Later in his practice, Freud saw persons with other psychological problems, such as phobias and obsessive-compulsive preoccupations. These individuals were similar to hysterics in that they complained of discrete, unwanted, and disturbing experiences. They differed from hysterics in that their "symptoms" did not resemble neurological disease. Freud also classified these persons as mentally ill and explained their neuroses by the same basic theories he used for hysteria.

The social context of psychiatry soon changed again. As the reputation of psychoanalysis spread, it was sought not only by persons who suffered from the discrete symptoms of the neuroses, but also by those who were experiencing disturbing problems in living and vague feelings of dissatisfaction and lack of fulfillment in their lives.[79] Also, increasing numbers of "normal" persons sought training analysis. Gradually, psychiatrists were invited to consult with social agencies, particularly the courts and the military services. These agencies asked psychiatrists to see persons who could be considered neither neurotic nor psychotic. Under these circumstances, the category of mental disease was broadened to include styles and patterns of conduct and character that had not previously been considered as diseases. The category of the "neurotic character" or "character disorder" was established for this purpose.[80]

As new categories of mental illness were created to justify expanding psychiatric functions, the differences from previous categories were ignored. Thus, over a period of time, such diverse phenomena as brain disease, depression, paranoia, sexual deviations, criminality, indolence, and the emotional crises of adolescence were included in the class of mental diseases. Indeed, all forms of human conduct can be considered as evidence of an underlying mental illness. The explanation for this is that the various "mental diseases" are basically similar because they have been ascribed to persons on whom psychiatric services have been performed.

The chart on page 109 illustrates the historical development of psychiatric nosology. The classification of each of these phenomena is superficially justified by its similarity to a preceding category. No single characteristic, however, is shared by each member of this group in the way, for instance, that all vertebrates from mouse to man, have rigid spinal

SOCIAL FUNCTION	DISEASE	SIMILARITY TO A PRECEDING CATEGORY ****	DIFFERENCE FROM A PRECEDING CATEGORY ****
Medical Practice	1. Medical disease		
Hospital Psychiatry	2. Organic brain disease	Caused by bodily disorder	Psychological symptoms prominent
	3. Psychosis	Disabling psychological symptoms requiring hospitalization	No organic basis
Office Practice (Psychoanalysis and psychotherapy)	4. Conversion hysteria	Resembles bodily disease	No actual bodily disease
	5. Other psycho-neurosis	Discrete "symptoms"; psychological conflict; undesirable	No resemblance to physical disease
Social Psychiatry	6. Character neurosis; behavioral malad-justments	Psychological conflict; undesirable	Patterned behavior rather than discrete symptoms

columns. This can be seen most clearly by comparing the first member of the group with the last, by comparing organic brain disease with character neurosis. What is the similarity between a hard driving executive who is also dependent on his wife, and a man with cancer or senile brain disease? What are the similarities between a mongoloid child and a presidential assassin? This illustrates the main similarity between the members of the class of illness—all are considered in one way or another to represent undesirable states. The main similarity between the members of the class of mental illness is that they are the objects of psychiatric attention. The differentiation of one category of mental illness from another is the result primarily of the historical differentiation of the social functions of psychiatry, rather than the logical refinement of the concept of mental illness.

PSYCHIATRY, "MENTAL ILLNESS," AND SOCIAL VALUES

To place psychiatry in a proper social perspective, it is necessary to consider two propositions about mental illness. First, there is the proposition, that mental illness is a label ascribed by psychiatrists to persons whom they wish to mark as deviant, to control, and to influence. A corollary of this proposition is that if one wishes to understand mental illness, one must understand the social functions of psychiatry.

The second proposition asserts that mental illness is more than a socially useful label: that mental illness refers to a process within certain individuals. A corollary of this proposition is that if one wishes to understand mental illness, one must study persons who exhibit its features.

To examine the second proposition closely is extremely important. Upon initial reflection, the two propositions may seem to be compatible. Indeed, many psychiatrists hold both propositions to be correct: that social values and conventions may influence the use of the concept "mental illness," but that this term also refers to an "objective" process that is independent of psychiatric values and operations. However, this view is false. The "objective" concept of mental illness has simply been abstracted from the social situations in which its meaning developed.[81] To claim that mental illness has a meaning independent of psychiatric social functions and values is analogous to claiming that money has a meaning outside of the economic system in which it is used. Moreover, the abstracted "objective" sense of the term "mental illness" still has a social utility, namely to disguise and distract us from the social functions of psychiatry. For the persistence of the view that mental illness has a meaning independent of the social functions of psychiatry leads, in practice, to the insistence, for any given use of the term, that the independent rather than the socially motivated meaning of the term is implied.

To obtain genuine, "objective, scientific determinations" of mental illness, it would have to be investigated in laboratory circumstances, divorced and insulated from personal and social values and interests. This is the meaning of the words "objective" and "disinterested" as they characterize research in the physical sciences. Such an investigation, however, is clearly impossible because human behavior, unlike physical events, cannot be understood except in the context of social conventions and cannot be evaluated except in the context of social values. Social science, including psychiatric, research cannot be disinterested nor objective and therefore cannot be scientific in the same sense as the physical and biological sciences.

For those mental processes supposedly unique to the mentally ill to be known, they must be disruptive enough for the person who experiences them to come to the attention of a psychiatrist, either voluntarily or against his will. What an individual does or experiences before he sees a psychiatrist has occurred and can be described. Only when he has seen a psychiatrist, however, can these occurrences be "authoritatively" labelled as mental illness. The identification of these processes as illnesses is therefore immutably linked to the processes by which persons are brought to the attention of psychiatrists; these, in turn, are linked to the social functions of psychiatry.

If the psychiatrist is a private therapist whose role is to analyze his patients, the question of mental illness need not arise because it is not instrumental to the goals of therapy. The determining factors of a patient's entry into psychotherapy are that he wants it and can pay for it, not that he has mental illness and is in need of treatment. If the psychiatrist functions to confine individuals or to control and manage their behavior, he must use the concept of mental illness to justify his interventions. Once a person is seen by a psychiatrist, the explanations given for the patient's thoughts, feelings, and actions are given in the social context of psychiatric operations to manipulate and control him or to understand him.[82]

We must distinguish between knowledge about the concept of "mental illness" and knowledge about the behavior given this label. The social matrix of *the concept of mental illness* is equivalent to the social matrix of psychiatry. The social matrix of the *behavior labelled as mental illness* is equivalent to the social matrix of that person's life. The concepts of mental health and illness are not necessary to understand human behavior; they have a social not a scientific utility.

While we do not require the concepts of health and illness to understand an individual, we do require a knowledge of social and moral conventions. Attempts to explain the behavior of persons labelled as mentally ill are no different than attempts to explain the behavior of persons labelled as mentally healthy. The task in both cases is the explanation of human conduct. The behavior of persons labelled as mentally ill may be unusual, puzzling, and bizarre and therefore more difficult to explain. This, however, is not because of a special and distinct mental process in these individuals. Human behavior is explained in terms of social conventions, and familiar (or conventional) behavior is more easily understood than unfamiliar (or unconventional) behavior.[83] In the case of unfamiliar (and therefore, deviant) behavior, an additional name for that behavior, such as mental illness, is not required, nor is the presumption of a special process which lies behind and causes it. A deeper inquiry into the motives, strategies, styles and life situation of the individual involved is required. Such an inquiry will usually reveal that this person is pursuing conventional goals in an extraordinary fashion, that he is using ordinary means in the pursuit of unusual or unconventional goals, or that he has imaginatively and metaphorically interpreted his life experiences in a manner that, although it may differ from most people's, is nevertheless quite understandable.[84]

Persons labelled as mentally ill are distinguished from other persons on two grounds—they have been *labelled* as mentally ill and they may have exhibited behavior judged to be deviant, enigmatic, or undesirable. On the *basis* of these distinctions, special mental processes are often postulated to lie behind and *cause* these differences. These special processes are then used to mark the mentally ill as a special group on (allegedly) scientific, as well as on social grounds. However, this scientific theorization functions to justify viewing the "mentally ill" as a different kind of human being, whom we may therefore treat differently from the "mentally healthy," for instance, by making them exceptions to constitutional guarantees and to the Rule of Law.

There is thus a serious question of whether the "scientific" search for *pathological* mental processes serves social rather than scientific purposes. There is evidence to suggest, for instance, that socially useful and even virtuous conduct as well as socially deviant and harmful conduct are associated with these alleged "pathological" processes. For instance, scientists are often obsessively concerned with their life's work, and they are usually compulsive about procedures, precautions, and details involving this work. Artists often fantasy and daydream, and they often claim that their work is the result of an unconscious "process" over which they have no control. Indeed, "normal" persons are often automatically obedient to social norms, rules, and laws to a degree that they could be considered not to be in control of their actions. As long as the behavior of these persons is considered to be socially desirable and useful, they are not defined as mentally ill and confined in psychiatric hospitals or forced to receive psychotherapy. The "mentally ill" person is not marked off from others by his hidden "pathological" mental processes. He is marked off by the fact that social and psychiatric authorities wish to stigmatize, deface and control his conduct.[85] To disguise this motive, they postulate special mental processes that it is their intention to "treat."

The concept of mental illness therefore represents a group ideal as a means to measure and evaluate an individual's social performance. It is possible to sketch in general terms the social values upon which the distinction between mental health and illness is based in our society.[86]

Included among these values are a commitment and loyalty to social groups—the family, the collective, and the nation. Also included are prevalent moral and legal codes of conduct, particularly the respect of community tranquility and safety. These values are also materialistic and worldly and involve an interest in goods, productivity, thrift, industry, and prudence. Also, they contain elements of Christian asceticism—self-control and the moderation of sensual pleasures, particularly of sexual pleasures. Finally, they include whatever modes of thought and conduct conform to the standards of those with social power and influence.

From this point of view, to label a person as mentally ill is simply to mark his deviation from one or another of these standards, rather than to describe and explain his conduct. It labels him as bad, it justifies his isolation from the group, it classifies him as in need of behavioral and thought reform, and it deprives his actions of social legitimacy. If one were to examine the "case" histories of mentally ill persons, it would be an easy task to identify the conventions and morals from which they have deviated, upon which the label of mental illness was based, and it would be simple, on this basis, to predict the goals to which psychiatric therapy would set itself.

PART TWO

The Social Functions of Psychiatry

CHAPTER FIVE

Involuntary Psychiatric Hospitalization

> . . . a purpose that cannot fully stand the light of scrutiny expresses itself in a form suitable to other purposes: aggressive acts of individuals and social groups often drape themselves in the mantle of morality, and the declared purpose is often not the real one.
>
> —CHARLES W. MORRIS[1]

The mental hospital is the historical and functional keystone of psychiatry, and involuntary hospitalization is its most important function. The influence and power of the mental hospital reach to most other psychiatric activities, and the clinical and scientific rhetoric of psychiatry are designed to support its purposes.

THE PSYCHIATRIC HOSPITAL AND THE MEDICAL MODEL

The term "psychiatric hospital" immediately prejudices one to think of mental institutions according to the medical model. The inmates are thought of as "patients," who suffer from "mental diseases" and receive "care and treatment" from "doctors and nurses." In the details of rhetoric and decor, we are invited to think of the psychiatric hospital as a medical installation.

Important differences exist, however, between psychiatric and medical hospitals. The most conspicuous is that a person may be involuntarily admitted to and detained in a psychiatric hospital but not a medical hospital. Involuntary detention is usually more closely associated with social control than with medical treatment, and houses of detention are more usually called prisons than hospitals. Why then is involuntary psychiatric hospitalization conceptualized within the framework of medical treatment rather than within the framework of social control?

This question cannot be answered by an examination of psychiatric language nor by an analysis of the expressed explanations and motives of psychiatrists. For such an examination will reveal only that psychiatrists prefer the language of medicine to describe and justify their practice. The question must be answered by comparing psychiatric commitment with *operations* that are paradigmatic of medical treatment and of social control. The test of whether the medical model or the social control model better fits the mental hospital must begin with a comparison of the *social situations* of the involuntary psychiatric patient, the hospitalized medical patient (the paradigm of medical treatment) and the imprisoned criminal (the paradigm of social control). Then must be considered the point of view or purpose underlying the present tendency to classify the involuntary mental patient with the medical patient in the context of medicine.

A COMPARISON OF THE SOCIAL SITUATIONS OF
INMATES OF PSYCHIATRIC, MEDICAL
AND PENAL INSTITUTIONS

*Comparison of the Social Circumstances
of Entrance into the Institution*

There is general agreement in our culture about the value of a long life, free of pain and diminished bodily function.

Most persons willingly seek medical treatment, including hospital treatment, when it is deemed to be necessary. However, a physically ill adult (who is not an inmate of a total institution) may refuse to enter a hospital without fear of being coerced to do so, except when the health of the public is placed in jeopardy, as in the case of special contagious diseases. In these special situations, the legal action to require treatment is clearly defined as for the benefit of the community. Medical hospitalization and treatment may be undertaken without a patient's consent if he is unconscious; for the physician to continue treatment, however, it is mandatory that the patient's consent be obtained once he has regained consciousness. Medical treatment may also be undertaken without a patient's consent if he is a member of a total institution, for instance a prison or the armed forces. In these situations, however, those who call for the treatment have clear and legitimate social power over the patient. This social power, rather than "scientific" or "medical" claims about the nature of the patient's illness, justifies the coercive treatment.

If an individual rejects medical treatment, his family may force it upon him by petitioning for a declaration of mental incompetence. His family's consent will then be legally sufficient to have that person treated in either a medical or a psychiatric hospital. This illustrates a primary difference between the medically ill and the mentally ill: namely, that the former cannot be forced to accept treatment against their will unless they are converted to the status of mental patients, who can be hospitalized and treated without their consent. Consistent with this, there are no facilities in this country for treating involuntary *medical* patients outside of a total institution, while most *mental* hospitals contain involuntary patients.

The majority of psychiatric patients are hospitalized against their will. In New York State in 1960, for example, only slightly more than one-fifth of state mental hospital admissions were voluntary.[2] However, the word "involuntary" is misleading, since any of these patients could be retained in the hospital against his will and be converted to an involuntary status.[3]

The admission of physically ill persons to medical hospitals is relatively simple. All that such persons need do is to present themselves to a physician at a hospital, clinic, office, or home. The physician who believes that the patient's condition warrants it will arrange his entrance into the hospital. The patient must give his consent for treatment, but he need not agree to remain in the hospital for any specified period of time, and he may change physicians when he pleases. Court hearings are not required and problems of civil rights rarely arise.

The situation is quite different in the case of the mental patient. In New York State, recent legislation has provided five different routes of admission. Only one of these routes is at all similar to that of the medical patient—the so-called informal admission. A patient admitted on an informal basis need not agree to remain in the hospital for any specified period, and he may leave the hospital when he wishes, provided that it is during "business" hours and provided that the hospital authorities do not seek "another form of admission." The informal admission is usually viewed with disfavor by hospital psychiatrists who object to the burden of processing patients who leave shortly after arriving. One explicit motive for the informal admission is that it makes entrance into a mental hospital similar to entrance into a medical hospital. However, this is only a "token" reform. In the few states having this type of admission, it is of recent origin and rarely used.

The second form of admission to the mental hospital is the so-called "voluntary." In this case, the patient agrees to stay in the hospital for fifteen days, but may be detained for an additional ten days at the discretion of the hospital director. If the director does not wish to discharge the patient then, he may request court authorization to detain him further. The court may order such a patient to be confined for a period not to exceed six months the first time, up to twelve months the second time, and up to twenty-four months thereafter.

The third form of admission is for the patient who does not, of his own initiative, seek an informal or voluntary admission, but who does not object to hospitalization. Such a patient may be admitted upon the certification of one physician. He may be detained up to fifteen days, whereupon either he must be converted to voluntary status, or a second physician's certificate must be obtained. From that time on, such an inmate will be treated as if he were admitted by the fourth route—the two physician certificate. This form of certification is for an individual who is unwilling to comply with the wishes of others that he enter a mental institution. Such a person may be detained for up to sixty days, following which he must be discharged, converted to an informal or voluntary status, or further detained by court authorization.

The fifth admission route is by means of the Health Officer's Certificate. Any individual who, in the opinion of a Commissioner of Health, County Health Officer, Director of Community Mental Health Services, or a designee approved by the Department of Mental Hygiene, is dangerous to himself or to others or is in need of immediate care for mental illness, may be committed to a psychiatric hospital for a period of up to fifteen days. After this period, the patient must be discharged, converted to an informal or voluntary status, or be detained by means of a two physician certificate.

This procedure means, in effect, that government health officials may deprive any individual of freedom without bail for fifteen days or longer by certifying that he is dangerous to himself or to others, or that he is in need of psychiatric treatment. Unlike the medically ill individual who may refuse to be hospitalized, any person who is accused of being mentally ill may be deprived of his freedom by means of involuntary psychiatric hospitalization. The requirement for one or two physician's certificate is not an overwhelming obstacle since there are usually physicians in every community who are willing to perform this service.

Many persons who realize that they are vulnerable to psychiatric power will admit themselves to psychiatric hospitals on an informal or voluntary basis to avoid stronger coercion. Such persons are often euphemistically referred to by junior psychiatric staff as "involuntary voluntaries." In one instance a woman was brought to a psychiatric hospital bound and tied by her husband and mother-in-law. In spite of her unwillingness to receive psychiatric "treatment" she signed a voluntary admission form to avoid the threatened alternative of involuntary hospitalization. Such circumstances are not reflected in the statistics for informal and voluntary admissions.

A major similarity between the criminal and the mental patient is that both are deprived of their freedom against their will. Both differ from the hospitalized medical patient in this respect. However, the allegedly mentally ill person who is being considered for commitment does not enjoy the same legal protections as the accused criminal. Under the old New York State Mental Hygiene Law, a prospective mental patient was entitled to a court hearing before certification. However, the Special Committee to Study Commitment Procedures of the Association of the Bar of New York City admitted that ". . . the vast majority of patients certified to State hospitals under Section 74 [two physician certificate] receive no hearing, and many do not even receive a notice indicating that they are entitled to a hearing."[4]

The revised New York State Law establishes a Mental Health Information Service that is supposed to inform involuntary mental patients of their legal rights. These rights, however, are meager compared to those enjoyed by the criminal. Judicial certification hearings have been omitted, and the confined mental patient is entitled to a hearing only after he has been committed and labelled as mentally ill and then only in four circumstances: (1) upon a writ of habeus corpus submitted in his behalf; (2) upon the request of the patient, a relative, a friend, or the Mental Health Information Service; (3) before the expiration period of sixty days for a patient committed involuntarily; and (4) before the expiration period of six months, one year, or two years after a previously authorized court retention.

On the other hand, before a criminal is confined, he is entitled to the right to sufficient notice, the right to counsel, the right to be presented with a specific written bill, the right to be confronted by his accusers, the right to trial by jury in an adversary proceeding, the right to refuse to bear witness against himself, and the right to appeal.

Although mental patients have the right to legal representation, most of them are too poor to afford it, and usually they are not assigned lawyers by the court. Indeed, they are often prevented from appearing at their own hearing on the grounds that it would be unduly psychologically disturbing for them. This decision is made by the psychiatrists who will testify against them!

The accused criminal must defend himself against a written bill of facts; the accused mental patient must defend himself against psychiatric testimony that he is mentally ill, potentially dangerous, and in need of care and treatment. This testimony is presented in vague, pseudoscientific language so flexible that it may be used against anyone. Nor is the commitment hearing an adversary procedure. The psychiatrists who testify against the allegedly mentally ill person are employed by the state, which is a party to the decision. Yet, these psychiatrists are considered to be "neutral" experts. This is comparable to having the prosecuting attorney in a criminal trial testify as an expert against the defendant! Moreover, the "mentally ill" defendant may engage a psychiatrist to testify in his behalf only if he has the funds, which often, he does not have.

The information presented by the psychiatric "expert" witness in his testimony against the patient-defendant is obtained from that patient during the course of what is supposed to be a confidential doctor-patient relationship. Thus, the defendant in a commitment hearing is not protected from testifying against himself. On the contrary during interviews with the hospital psychiatrist, the defendant supplies the bulk of the evidence against himself. Refusal to cooperate with the psychiatrist, rather than being within his rights under the Fifth Amendment, may be construed as evidence for a "paranoid illness" for which he requires further psychiatric hospitalization.[5]

A 1967 Supreme Court decision recognized that juvenile defendants are entitled to the same constitutional protections as adults—to protections against unreasonable arrest, search and seizure; to the right to adequate written notice; to the right to be represented by counsel; and to the right not to bear witness against oneself. This decision leaves involuntary psychiatric patients as the only group not receiving these constitutional protections.

In his opinion in this case, Justice Fortas stated:

> A boy is charged with misconduct. The boy is committed to an institution where he may be restrained of liberty for years. It is of no constitutional consequence —and of limited practical meaning—that the institution to which he is committed is called "an industrial school." The fact of the matter is that, however euphemistic the title, a "receiving home" or an "industrial school" for juveniles is an institution of confinement. His world becomes a building with whitewashed walls, regimented routine and institutional law.[6]

The same is true of persons who are involuntarily confined in mental hospitals; one need only replace the words "misconduct" and "industrial school" with "mental illness" and "mental hospital."

The legal safeguards afforded to the criminal are considered by most psychiatrists as "legal encumbrances" that would stigmatize and distress the mental patient and delay his access to "medical" care. Thus, the rationale behind the commitment laws in New York State is given as being ". . . to place mentally ill persons on a par with other sick persons, and make available to them . . . hospitalization in medical treatment facilities."[7] This legislation was inspired by a committee of lawyers who advocated that: "When a person must be sent to a mental hospital against his will, he should not be treated like a criminal and be tried and convicted of being sick."[8]

This rhetoric, however, requires critical examination; it overlooks the fact that the involuntarily hospitalized mental patient differs from "other" sick persons and resembles the criminal in that he is confined against his will. No other social group so closely resembles the criminal in this respect. The abandonment of legal safeguards—the direction taken by recent "liberal" mental health legislation—serves primarily to disguise this resemblance. This results in the irony that while the involuntary incarceration of the criminal is defined as punitive, it is defined as helpful for the mental patient, and while the traditional constitutional safeguards against the loss of liberty are defined as helpful to the criminal, they are defined as harmful to the mental patient.

Comparison of the Social Circumstances of Institutional Living

The social situation of the institutionalized mental patient more closely resembles that of the imprisoned criminal than it does that of the hospitalized medical patient. Both the hospitalized mental patient and the confined criminal are inmates of total institutions. A total institution is defined by Erving Goffman as ". . . a place of residence and work where a large number of like situated individuals, cut off from the wider society for an appreciable period of time, together lead an enclosed, formally administered round of life."[9]

Mental hospitals and prisons may be classified as total institutions to the extent that they exhibit the following features.[10]

(1) *There is a status split and little intimate contact between the staff and the inmates.*

It is likely that the mental hospital inmate will belong to a lower socioeconomic class than will his hospital psychiatrist.[11] However, the primary obstacle to their intimacy and the main difference in their status is due to the social power the psychiatrist holds over his patient. The psychiatrist not only has the power to determine whether and when his patient will be released, but also to determine the nature of the patient's institutional life. Their relationship is thus often permeated with fear and suspicion and may be construed as antagonistic.[12] This power differential does not exist between a medical doctor and his private patient, first because they may be from the same social class and second, because the patient may fire his physician, hire another, and refuse to follow any medical directive.

(2) *A part of the daily routine consists of compulsory labor for which substandard remuneration is received.*

No matter how physically capable he may be, a patient in a medical hospital is not required to make his own bed, to clean his room, or to contribute to the housekeeping and upkeep of the hospital. Janitorial and nursing aid services are employed for this purpose. On the other hand, the inmates of prisons and of most mental hospitals are required to perform these tasks. In some mental institutions patients are made to care for the buildings and grounds and to work in kitchens, laundries, shops and offices. This forced labor is justified as a form of "occupational therapy" that will help the patient adjust to the world of work. This demonstrates that what is wrong with the medical patient is an improper functioning of his body, while one of the things "wrong" with the criminal and the mental patient is they do not engage in "responsible" work.

(3) *The family structure is fractured with relatively little contact between family members over a long time.*

To some small degree, the community psychiatry movement has eliminated this feature of the total psychiatric institution. The construction of new mental hospitals in urban rather than rural areas, the establishment of day and night care centers, the reduction of the length of confinement, and the increase of freedom of movement have enabled the inmates of some mental hospitals to maintain a semblance of contact with their family and community.

The inmates of large, rurally-located mental hospitals, however, are still separated from their families. This type of mental hospital is by far the more common. In this sense, the mental hospital more closely resembles the prison than the medical hospital, which is to be found primarily in urban and suburban locations.

Medical illness tends to mobilize and consolidate the family around the ill person, and visitors have easy access to patients in a medical hospital. However, both mental illness and criminality tend to fragment the family. Not only is the institutionalized mental patient physically removed from his family, but also often his conflict with his family has led *them* to petition for his commitment. Indeed, the community psychiatry movement has been spurred into existence by the dislocation and alienation of mental patients from their families. This attempt to overcome the results of family fragmentation is certainly proof of its existence.

(4) *There is a loss of self-determination in one's personal and social existence.*

To the extent that he is physically able, the patient in a medical hospital may regulate his personal and social affairs and determine for himself his daily activities. In the mental hospital and the prison, on the other hand, the inmates are relatively regimented. The following passage from Goffman describes the round of life in the total institution:

> First, all aspects of life are conducted in the same place and under the same single authority. Second, each phase of the member's daily activity is carried on in the immediate company of a large batch of others, all of whom are treated alike and required to do the same thing together. Third, all phases of the day's activities are tightly scheduled, with one activity leading at a prearranged time into the next, the whole

sequence of activities being imposed from above by a
system of explicit formal rulings and a body of officials.
Finally, the various enforced activities are brought
together into a single rational plan purportedly designed to fulfill the official aims of the institution . . .

The handling of many human needs by the bureaucratic organization of whole blocks of people—whether
or not this is a necessary or effective means of social
organization in the circumstances—is the key fact of
total institutions.[13]

Inmates of medical hospitals are regulated by the conventional rules of social deportment and hospital routine. Hospital rules are enforced by the medical personnel and no special guards or watchmen are employed to supervise the
patients. In mental hospitals and prisons, on the other hand,
the main function of the hospital staff is to supervise and
regiment the inmates, and the majority of institutional employees perform this function.

An important function of prisons and mental hospitals
is the regimentation of the inmates to supervise and control
them. By forcing the inmates to surrender the self-regulation
of their conduct, the institutional authorities may accomplish
their secondary task of "rehabilitating" the inmates—of converting their antisocial conduct into behavior that conforms
and adapts to society.

In mental hospitals, the mental health of the inmates is
measured by the degree to which hospital authorities accomplish this regimentation. Thus, if a patient fits well with
the regulated round of collective life, he may be described
as cooperative, sociable, calm, friendly, and well-adjusted to
hospital routine. If he withdraws from the regimented group,
he may be described as seclusive, withdrawn, depressed,
paranoid, or uncooperative.

If a patient becomes involved in disputes with other
inmates, he is likely to be described as hostile, aggressive,
belligerent, dangerous, and refractory to treatment. Any dis-

play of behavior that deviates from the institutional ideal is considered ipso facto to be evidence of the patient's continuing mental illness for which additional confinement and more intensive treatment are required.

Recently, it has become fashionable in some mental hospitals to establish "patient governments" on the theory that the loss of self-regulation is bad for morale and that practice in self-regulation is good preparation for life outside the hospital. It is an illusion, however, that patient governments increase the self-determination of the individual mental hospital inmate. They tend to substitute self-imposed patient regimentation for regimentation by the hospital authorities. They thus usually accomplish the regimentation and control sought by the hospital authorities while providing the advantage of converting conflicts between patients and staff into conflicts among patients. So long as hospitals retain the power to grant or deny freedom to the patients and to invalidate any rule passed by the patient government, they retain the power to determine the nature of the inmates' institutional life and fate.

Patient governments do not reduce the totalitarianism of the mental hospital; they disguise it. They are thus in line with the modern tendency toward the technicalization and "democratization" of tyranny—the replacement of overt social power by the technology of social engineering and collectivized social control.[14]

(5) *The inmates are effectively rendered incapable (by social means) of managing certain features of their outside life.*

If he is physically able, the hospitalized medical patient may vote, marry, make contracts, and engage in all other financial and civil activities. By contrast, the inmates of prisons and mental hospitals may not. In some states, commitment to a mental hospital results in the loss of all civil rights. In others, certain rights are informally suspended without challenge.

This reflects the fact that the "trouble" with the medical patient is that he is not functioning properly as a physico-chemical machine, while the "trouble" with the mental patient and the prisoner is that they are not functioning properly as citizens. When a medical patient's body is a threat to the community—for instance, if he has a communicable disease—he is isolated from it by quarantine. When an individual's actions are a threat to the community —for instance if he exhibits dangerous thoughts or actions— he is isolated from the community by confinement, and during this period of confinement his right to participate in social and civil activities is suspended. This serves not only to protect society from him, but also to punish him for his transgressions. Thus, the mental patient and the prisoner are deprived not only of their freedom, but also of participation in civil affairs.

(6) *The inmates are repeatedly degraded, abused, and humiliated by the loss of privacy, loss of personal property, forced medical treatment, and forced obedience to the commands of institutional authority buttressed by punitive sanctions.*

To a certain degree, medical hospitalization results in the loss of privacy and personal property, and requires compliance with institutional authority. There is, however, no comparison of the degree to which this is experienced by the mental patient and the prisoner.

Although physical violence and neglect have not completely disappeared, the main sources of inhumanity in the modern mental hospital come from humiliation, coercion, and the loss of dignity. In large mental hospitals, patients are humiliated by being forced to surrender all of their personal possessions; by being photographed, and fingerprinted; by sleeping in large rooms with beds arranged in intimate proximity; by performing their daily toiletry without privacy, under the supervision of attendants; by having no choice of meals or hours of dining; by having their mail opened, read, and censored by the hospital authorities; by being forced to attend daily routine activities without being consulted about their wishes; by regimentation and surveillance during these activities; by being forced to ingest mind-altering drugs; and through all of this, by being subjected to the self-righteous and condescending attitudes of the staff members and sometimes, to threats and beatings at their hands.

The main similarity between the social circumstances of the patient in a medical hospital and his counterpart in the public psychiatric hospital is that the medical model is used to describe and explain both. Minor medical problems may be treated in the mental hospital, but the more difficult cases are usually transferred to the "hospital's" hospital or to a nearby medical facility. Instead of being classified as an ancillary service, this medical care is often defined as one of the central functions of the establishment in support of the claim that the psychiatric hospital is a medical facility.[15]

One class of medical patients—medically ill prisoners—is confined to a total institution. Their confinement, however, is determined by social factors rather than by the nature of their disease. In general, social rather than medical factors determine the kind of hospital to which a medical patient will go. For instance, to be a patient in a private hospital, a medically ill person must have the means to pay his hospital bill; to be a patient in a charity hospital, one must be indigent; to be a patient in a military hospital, one must be a member of the armed forces; to be a patient in a prison hospital, one must be a criminal and confined to a penal institution.[16]

From the private hospital to the prison hospital, the patient has a decreasing amount of power with respect to the hospital authorities. The medical patient in a private hospital is free to select his physician and to fire him if he is dissatisfied. He is free to consent to or refuse treatment, to socialize with members of the staff (or other patients) and to conduct his business, personal, and civic affairs. He is obliged to follow the rules of conduct of the hospital, but if he violates those rules, he is likely to be either discharged or converted to the status of a mental patient. (Unless, of course, he commits a crime and is arrested.)

The prisoner-medical patient, on the other hand, more closely resembles the mental patient than he does any of the other classes of medical patient. He is not free to select his physician nor to fire him. He may be forced to submit to medical treatment. He may not leave the hospital when he wishes, and if he violates the rules of the hospital, he will likely be punished by the institutional authorities. The prisoner-medical patient, unlike any other medical patient, but like the mental patient, is restricted to his ward by locked doors and/or guards whose function is to enforce the institution's code of conduct. If he escapes from the institution he will be pursued by the police and returned. This is true also of the committed mental patient, but not of the medical patient.

There is an important difference between the prisoner-medical patient and the involuntary mental patient that contrasts with their similarities: *While the prisoner-medical patient has lost his freedom on the basis of something other than the disease for which he is being treated, the mental patient has lost his freedom solely on the basis of his "illness."* This shows that the consequences of being labelled as mentally ill and confined to a mental institution are similar to being convicted of a crime and confined to prison.

Comparison of the Circumstances of Departure

If he is physically capable of leaving the hospital, the medical patient cannot be legally detained against his will (without converting him to the status of a mental patient). Both the mental patient and the criminal, on the other hand, may be detained even for life. The most important characteristic of the situation of the involuntary mental patient is that he cannot terminate his status at will. Even if he entered a mental hospital voluntarily, a person who cannot depart when he wishes must be considered an involuntary patient. The committed mental patient most closely resembles the prisoner and most markedly differs from the private medical patient in this respect.

When the medical patient is discharged, he may sever all ties with the hospital. Even if he returns for follow-up tests or aftercare, the hospital claims no jurisdiction over his social behavior. The criminal, on the other hand, is often discharged on parole, and, lest he be returned to prison, he must conform his conduct to more stringent regulations than must the ordinary citizen.

The involuntary mental patient is rarely released unconditionally. Even if he is an adult who is legally responsible, the mental patient is often discharged in the "custody" of a member of his family or a friend. If there is no one to assume custody, the patient may be confined indefinitely. In some states, the mental patient is forced to retain ties with the confining institution. He is obliged to report to its representatives regularly and to demonstrate his fitness to remain at liberty. This discharged status is also often referred to as "parole" or as "a trial visit."

Unlike the discharged medical patient, persons who have been released from mental hospitals and prisons are often stigmatized and treated with prejudice. They are often viewed not only as having inferior social identities, but also as possessing some hidden personality defect, which is only temporarily submerged and is likely to erupt again. On these grounds, discharged mental patients may be barred from employment; from military service; from acceptance to college; from holding public office; from entering into particular social circles; and in many states from exercising certain civil rights, such as the right to vote, to sue, to make contracts, to transfer property, and to testify.

Most public mental hospitals are overcrowded with patients and short of staff. It is possible to control inmates with a small staff, but not to treat them. Considering this, the refusal to discharge patients at their request and the conversion of voluntary patients to involuntary status raises some doubt that "treatment" is the primary concern.

The similarities between the social situations of hospitalized medical and mental patients fall into two categories—linguistic and procedural. The linquistic similarities cannot be considered crucial because they are derivatives of the fact that mental institutions are defined and classified as medical facilities in which medical services are performed. Since we are inquiring into the reasons for the medical classification of involuntary psychiatric hospitalization, we cannot consider the fact of that classification as an explanation for itself.

The procedural similarities are based on mental patients often being medicated and receiving other somatic treatments, such as shock therapy. Also, their medical ills are diagnosed and treated by hospital physicians. The question, however, is whether these medications and treatments perform primarily a physiological or a social function and whether the medical activities of hospital psychiatrists are to be considered central or ancillary.

There are important differences between the operations of medical and psychiatric physicians and between the social situations of medical and psychiatric patients. And there are important similarities between the situations of hospitalized mental patients and prisoners. What could be the purpose of classifying the hospitalized mental patient with the hospitalized medical patient in the context of medicine instead of with the prisoner in the context of social control?

The purpose of this classification is to provide paralegal control, disguised as benevolent medical treatment, of certain types of deviant behavior. This classification is necessary because to openly classify mental hospitals as agencies of social control would be in ostentatious violation of the Constitution, for their inmates have been deprived of their freedom without having been convicted, by due process, of violating the law.

Social Control and Individual Freedom Under Rule of Law

The mandate for the disguised control of certain forms of deviant behavior is deeply rooted in the social changes that produced modern society out of primitive and peasant communities. With the transformation from status to contract societies, a new consciousness of individual rights, freedom and dignity developed. The political essence of this transformation was the replacement of the absolute ruler by the elected representative and the replacement of Rule of Man by Rule of Law.

According to Friedrich Hayek, Rule of Law means:

> . . . that government in all its actions is bound by rules fixed and announced beforehand—rules which make it possible to foresee with fair certainty how the authority will use its coercive powers in given circumstances and to plan one's individual affairs on the basis of that knowledge . . . While every law restricts individual freedom to some extent by altering the means which people may use in the pursuit of their aims, under the Rule of Law the government is prevented from stultifying individual efforts by *ad hoc* action. Within the known rules of the game the individual is free to pursue his personal ends and desires, certain that the powers of government will not be used deliberately to frustrate his efforts.[17]

Rule of Law is the primary political protector of individual freedom. According to Hayek, adherence to this Rule distinguishes a free society from a totalitarian society. The Rule of Law has two functions: to establish limits on individual behavior for the benefit of the group, and to restrain the state in its exercise of power to control and regulate the individual.

The development of Rule of Law placed a strain on modern societies that the (simultaneous) development of psychiatry seems designed to relieve. The development of Rule of Law divided the codes regulating human conduct into two groups: rules codified in law that the state can enforce and those uncodified in law that the state cannot enforce. These uncodified rules are an extended catalog of unwritten, traditional guidelines of conduct based on religious morality, customs, conventions, etiquette, and folk styles.

There are no laws to insure the intelligibility of speech, the conformity of belief, the moderation of emotions, or the predictability of conduct. A man may talk jibberish, claim that he is Napoleon, cry without apparent cause, or cower from an imagined persecutor without fear of *legal* prosecution and penalty.

Although not prohibited by law, each of these actions violates informal standards of proper conduct and thus threatens the security, stability, and predictability of the social environment. There is thus, a built-in conflict between the desire for personal freedom under law and the desire for a stable, predictable social order. As Herbert Muller observed: "The essential conditions of freedom are uncertainty, instability, a measure of insecurity, a measure of disunity and disorder."[18] To a certain degree then, the goals of individual freedom and social stability are mutually limiting.[19] The greater the degree of individual freedom, the greater the tolerance of individual variation and unpredictability must be; the more secure the social order, the more the range of permissible behavior must be restricted.

The Public Mental Hospital as an
Instrument of Social Control

Although individual freedom and social order are mutually limiting, there are simultaneous mandates for respect for individual freedom under law and for a greater degree of social stability and conformity than is provided by law. Our nation was founded on the principles of human rights, individual freedom, and Rule of Law. In the spirit of our political system, deviance is defined by law, and those who are accused of crime are guaranteed protections against the unlimited and arbitrary use of power by the state by means of stipulated procedures of arrest, trial, and appeal.

On the other hand, we are a people, like other peoples, whose conduct is regulated also by custom, convention, morality, and prejudice. We impose and sanction standards of success, productivity, and conformity in personal conduct. We value domestic tranquility in an orderly and predictable social environment. While we value Rule of Law and the punishment of only those who have been convicted of crime, we are disturbed by more than lawlessness. Although not wishing to mark as criminals those who have not been accused and convicted of violating the law, we nevertheless demand protection against certain disturbing behavior that is not unlawful.

In a society ruled by law there are problems in controlling conduct that, while legal, violates certain social conventions and social tranquility. Due to the diminished power of the family, clan, and community, which formerly enforced these conventions, we lack the social machinery for this control. Because of the restraints placed on government by the Rule of Law, we lack the legal machinery for this control.

To be convincingly respectful of personal liberty, a nation must be governed by laws that are neither harsh nor restrictive, or *it must convey the image of being so governed.* To convey this image, it is useful for a portion of its social control apparatus to be visible and for another portion to be invisible or disguised. The practice of involuntary psychiatric hospitalization is well suited to the task of disguised social control.

By identifying with medicine, psychiatry may trade on the prestige and reputation of that honorable profession and with the sciences of physics and biology. By employing the allegedly value-free rhetoric of health and disease, psychiatrists may codify traditional standards and conventions of conduct in scientific sounding language. Persons whose conduct is socially and ethically desirable are labelled mentally healthy; persons whose conduct is socially and ethically undesirable are labelled mentally ill. This permits us to justify the detention of persons whose behavior is disturbing, dangerous, or unusual (but not illegal) under the rubric of benevolent medical treatment, rather than oppressive police action. By means of involuntary confinement, the mental hospital permits us to satisfy our desire to be protected from noncriminal deviations of conduct without suffering the guilt and embarrassment of violating our ideals of individual freedom under Rule of Law. The medical model permits us to control certain individuals under the guise of providing them with medical care, and it permits us to dismiss their objections to our coercion by explaining their protests as the madness of a mind that does not recognize that it is "ill.'"

To disguise a paralegal social control apparatus, the psychiatric hospital is classified in the context of medicine rather than in the context of social control.

THE STRUCTURE AND FUNCTION OF THE
MODERN MENTAL HOSPITAL

The primary function of the public mental hospital is to protect the community from persons whose conduct is considered to be dangerous, threatening, or bothersome. The physical and social structures of the mental hospital support this function and the rhetoric of medicine disguises it.

The physical structure of the mental hospital is designed to confine its inmates securely. The fenced grounds, the series of locked doors and elevators, the barred windows, the large open wards, the open toilet stalls, and the strategically located nurses' stations are all constructed to provide security and surveillance.

The social structure of the mental hospital is designed to perform the same function. In medical hospitals, the chief administrator is usually a civilian, and there is no pretense that his orders and rulings constitute medical treatment (although they may facilitate it). In mental hospitals, however, the chief administrator is a psychiatrist. This serves to justify confinement, security, and surveillance as medical activities. Any manipulation of the hospital environment may be justified as in the "therapeutic" interests of patients.[20] In effect, the use of psychiatrists rather than lay administrators permits social actions to be garbed as medical programs.

The mental hospital administrator autocratically rules a professional staff arranged in a strict hierarchy of authority. His primary concern is for hospital tranquility and security, the maintainence of which is often described as a milieu therapy program. When staff shortages do not permit individualized attention to patients, this milieu program is usually cited as the primary therapeutic service. In hospitals that have opened their doors, the lower echelon staff members are assigned such security functions as guarding exits and hallways and supervising patient groups.

Closely related to the primary function of the mental hospital as a place of confinement is its function as an instrument for modifying and correcting the thought and behavior of its inmates. (In medical rhetoric, this function is described as providing care and treatment for mentally ill patients.) All of the methods available to modern man for influencing men's minds — confinement, regimentation, propaganda, threats, punishment, humiliation, bribes, drugs, and physical manipulations—are applied to this purpose. The most important tool available to the hospital psychiatrist, however, is his social power over the inmate to continue or end his confinement and to regulate his institutional life. Of course, when these methods are described with the medical model, they have the appearance of modern, humane techniques of "psychological" medicine.

More broadly conceived, three additional functions of the public mental hospital are of social significance and deserve brief mention.

First, the use of the mental hospital to confine, control, supervise, and reform deviant individuals is a device for circumventing the restraint that Rule of Law places on the power of the state. The fact that psychiatrists describe the functions of the public mental hospital in terms of benevolent medical motives does not alter this. In a society ruled by law, social actions must be judged according to the standards and ideals of law rather than according to supralegal ideals and values. In the sense that psychiatric commitment accomplishes an unconstitutional act—confinement without trial—it is a violation of and a form of disobedience to the constitution condoned by the whole society.

We tend to think of civil disobedience as only a protest by a minority against laws it considers unfair and inequitable. Civil disobedience, however, may also be used by the majority to protest or circumvent laws that are inconvenient or unpopular. Disobedience of the Volstead Act was of such a nature. Alcohol is extremely popular in this country, and the Eighteenth Amendment was widely violated until it was repealed. The repeal of the Eighteenth Amendment to the Constitution, however, had no deep significance for our political structure and ideals.

The Bill of Rights and the Rule of Law place such severe restrictions on government's capacity to control and regulate behavior that the State itself has participated in practices that circumvent these restraints. In this sense, psychiatric commitment may be viewed as a form of disobedience to the most fundamental and political principles and instruments of our society. This evasion must be disguised in the rhetoric of medicine because we are apt neither to repeal the Bill of Rights nor to recognize openly the inconvenience it causes us in our efforts to control and regulate conduct.

A second function of the mental hospital is therefore to protect our image as a free society, devoted to Rule of Law. It permits us to hide violations of the principle of individual freedom under law in order to improve our internal security and tranquility. The image of our nation as a free society would be badly tarnished if it were openly recognized that an individual could be confined without trial, bail, or due process by means of psychiatric commitment. Such a revelation could easily be used as propaganda against us by our adversaries in the Cold War, with whom our main ideological difference is that their societies are closed (lack individual freedoms) and ours is open.[21] Psychiatry thus serves nationalistic and patriotic, rather than medical and scientific, causes.

A third social function of psychiatric commitment is that it serves as a supplement to and a replacement of the extended family for the purpose of regulating and controlling individual behavior. Psychiatric commitment serves to buttress and support the unstable nuclear family. Where extended family structures are preserved and viable, conduct is regulated primarily by this group, and deviants are usually managed within the group rather than by expulsion.[22] Psychiatry develops as an institution where extended family structures tend to break down into nuclear groups—for instance in urban and industrial areas. It helps the family control and correct the conduct of deviant persons. Functionally, therefore, the psychiatric hospital is a supplement to and a replacement for the extended family.

Most of the inmates of mental hospitals have been committed as the result of a petition by a family member. Psychiatric commitment is often the result of an acute or prolonged family disruption, which results in the exclusion and isolation of one member (usually the least powerful). Psychiatric commitment therefore serves to relieve intolerable family conflicts by removing one member from the group.

The medical rhetoric of psychiatry permits this expulsion to be defined as a benevolent and sympathetic action taken for the benefit of the family member who is "ill" and "in need of treatment." This terminology facilitates the subsequent reintegration and reconciliation of the discharged member into the family. Indeed, much of the little hospital therapy provided aims at the restoration of family relationships. If it were not for the psychiatric rhetoric, the petition for commitment of one family member by another would be recognized as explicitly punitive and antagonistic, as is reporting to the police a relative who has committed a crime. The medical model thus relieves the family of the embarrassment and guilt of betraying a family member, and it encourages the expelled member to reconcile himself with gratitude to the fact that his family acted in his own best interests.

Involuntary confinement is by far the most important function of the modern mental hospital. However, some mental hospitals admit voluntary patients who are permitted to leave when they wish. Some comments should be made about voluntary mental hospitalization, lest it be presumed that such hospitalization, where it exists, serves a medical rather than a social function.

Theoretically, the voluntary mental hospital could provide an opportunity for escape and renewal for persons who are unprepared for or overwhelmed by the stresses and strains of modern life. Persons who are wealthy rarely use the public mental hospital for this purpose; they use the luxurious private asylum and hotel instead.

The function of the voluntary hospital is generally equivalent to the function of religious retreats, vacations and travel. Each of these activities provides an adult social moratorium: a period of relief from responsibility and obligations. One may rest, relax, enjoy food prepared by others, read, reflect, and engage in pleasant conversation. There is an opportunity to review one's life, to reformulate plans and strategies, and to rededicate one's self for reentering the fray.

In our society, an individual may not simply call a moratorium on his social responsibilities unless he is extremely wealthy. He is expected to work, to fulfill his social obligations, and to meet head on whatever difficulties and strains he encounters in the process. The only time an individual may legitimately suspend his duties and obligations is when he is ill and has been so certified by a physician.[23] Illness may be used as an excuse from work, from school, from military service, from being executed, and from discharging any civic duty.

The patient in a mental hospital, however, is not physically ill. He suffers from problems in living, not from disease. He may be in unbearable conflict with his family, friends, or employer; he may be experiencing difficulty at work, at school, or in his social relations; he may be in financial or sexual trouble; he may be unsure of the purpose and meaning of life; or he may be encountering one of the multitude of other problems that are a part of being alive.

By using the metaphor of illness to describe these problems, it is possible for persons who are not wealthy to suspend their ordinary activities without beng accused of irresponsibility, immorality, cowardice, or some other social weakness. Instead, they may be regarded sympathetically, as the victims of some natural disease beyond their powers to prevent and for which they require hospitalization and treatment.

By providing a socially acceptable disguise, the medical model facilitates a voluntary social moratorium for the middle and lower classes. An opportunity for such a moratorium may be an advantage in a complex, stressful society such as ours. The medical model, however, creates the disadvantage of influencing the voluntary patient to view his problems in the context of illness and health rather than in the context of ethics, psychology, economics, politics, and social relations. It thus handicaps his efforts to understand and deal intelligently with his troubles. Also, the institutionalized helpers with whom these patients come into contact are, for the most part, trained in medicine and are not always well prepared to understand and interpret the dilemmas of persons who are plagued by problems in living.[24] Finally, the public mental hospitals into which these troubled persons enter deal primarily with the involuntary patient. The needs of the voluntary patient are subordinated to this function.

INSTITUTIONS FOR THE MENTAL DEFECTIVE

In every society there are persons who cannot (or do not) discharge their social responsibilities and who are therefore labelled as incapable or inept. In primitive and peasant communities, such persons may be kept within the group, given some simple tasks to perform, and be cared for by members of their families or village. It is very likely that there are fewer defectives in simple societies because most individuals can perform tasks that satisfy the demands of the group for a contribution. Complex societies will produce more social judgments of mental defectiveness because greater skills are required for transacting normal social and economic activities. In advanced urban societies, where the integrity of the clan and extended family are disrupted and where the work is specialized, the family is often unable and unwilling to accept the burden of caring for these persons. Special institutions have therefore been constructed by the state for this purpose. Institutions for the mental defective are somewhat different from the ordinary mental hospital and thus require separate consideration.

In general, there are two types of mental deficiency. One type is caused by demonstrable physical diseases, such as mongolism or congenital brain deformity, which alters the structure and function of the brain and is associated with low intelligence. For the most part, these diseases are incurable and primarily require nursing and custodial care. For these people, therefore, institutions for mental defectives function more like nursing homes than like ordinary medical hospitals.

A second type of mental deficiency cannot be associated with demonstrable physical disease, although sometimes such disease is presumed to exist. The sole basis for the confinement of these individuals is, allegedly, their low intelligence, on which basis they are often detained from early childhood until death. Defective intelligence is classified as a mental disease. The institutions in which mental defectives are confined are staffed by physicians and are often referred to as hospitals.

The standard index of mental deficiency is intelligence, which, as everyone knows, is measured by intelligence tests. Intelligence tests are viewed as psychological instruments for examining a person's mental status. It is assumed that they tell us something about the functioning of a person's mind in the same way, for instance, that an electrocardiogram tells us about the functioning of his heart. However, when we make a judgment about a person's intelligence we are not evaluating a ghostly process that goes on in his head; we are evaluating his *behavior* by judging it to be skillful, clumsy, slow, efficient, accurate, or erroneous in various ways. Intelligence is not something in addition to behavior, like a right hand glove is something in addition to a left hand glove. "Intelligence" is a comment about behavior in much the way that "pair" is a comment about two gloves. "The difference between a normal person and an idiot," says Gilbert Ryle, "is not that the normal person is two persons [a body and a mind] while the idiot is only one, [a body], but that the normal person can do a lot of things which the idiot cannot do."[25] (Brackets added.)

Mental defectiveness is not an isolated quality of an individual's brain or mind; it is a judgment that he does not or cannot perform desirable and prescribed activities. Like the person labelled mentally ill, the defective is usually committed because he causes problems for his family and his community. He is considered to be unable to achieve minimum standards of self-care and deportment and is judged to be a nuisance, a threat, or a burden.

However, moral and legal problems, which are rarely discussed, are associated with the involuntary confinement of mental defectives. The constitutional guarantees of freedom and due process are not reserved for only those who demonstrate normal intelligence, and subnormal intelligence is not a crime. In a society that cherishes individual freedom and Rule of Law, what is to be done with persons who demonstrate ineptness, clumsiness, an inability to solve ordinary social and intellectual problems, a continued failure to learn the rules of social deportment, and an inability to find and perform productive work?

The solution devised for this problem is to classify these persons as lacking intelligence, to classify the lack of intelligence as a disease, and to confine these persons in public institutions with the explanation that they are ill and in need of care and treatment. The classifications are called "scientific" and supported by "objective" tests that purport to measure the ineffable quality of intelligence. The moral, social, and legal aspects of the problem are thus disguised.

In this context, the intelligence test is a social tool, which, by passing as an objective, value-neutral, scientific measurement, may be used to justify the involuntary confinement of persons whose behavior is threatening, disturbing, or unconventional. In New York State, any person with a tested intelligence quotient of 80 or below may be legally confined in an institution for mental defectives. Of course, not all persons with an I.Q. below 80 are confined. This demonstrates that low intelligence is not the issue, but rather the violation of behavioral conventions. If a person is labelled as mentally ill, his I.Q. will simply determine whether he is committed to an institution for mental defectives or to an ordinary mental hospital.

Institutions for mental defectives are simply variations of the public mental hospital. They are used to confine a special class of undesirables: those who are considered to be incapable of caring for themselves and of adequately discharging their social obligations. As in the case of the public mental hospital, the medical model is used to disguise the social and ethical issues involved and to justify a solution to a problem that, if it were viewed in social and political terms, would be much more difficult to resolve. It would be difficult to establish a rule of law governing general standards of social performance below which an individual could be deprived of his freedom for life. The problem is all the more difficult because the persons who are confined in this situation are the weakest elements in society, who are under the greatest pressure to surrender their freedom, and who have the least capacity to defend their rights. It is far simpler to disguise the problem as medical and psychiatric in nature and to leave it to the "medical experts" to solve.

CHAPTER SIX

Psychotherapy

Indeed, these words, "a secular spiritual guide" might well serve as a general formula for describing the function which the analyst, whether he is a doctor or a layman, has to perform in his relation to the public.

—SIGMUND FREUD[1]

Psychotherapy is often defined as the medical treatment of emotional and personality disorders by psychological means.[2] Even when psychotherapy is not explicitly classified as a medical technique, medical language is often used to describe and explain it. For instance, psychotherapy is often described as a *healing* art and science in which a *therapist* undertakes to *treat* a *patient* whose complaints are called *symptoms* for the purpose of *curing* or palliating his *illness*.

There is not consensus, however, that psychotherapy is a medical activity. For instance, Shoben defines it as: ". . . a certain kind of social relationship between two persons who hold periodic conversations in pursuit of certain goals: namely, the lessening of emotional discomfort and the alteration of various other aspects of client behavior."[3] Others explicitly deny that psychotherapy is, or ought to be, classified as a medical practice.[4]

Many persons believe the main significance of the medical-nonmedical nature of psychotherapy controversy is who should be permitted to practice psychotherapy. If psychotherapy is a medical activity, then it should be practiced only by physicians. If it is not a medical activity, then it may be practiced by qualified psychologists, social workers and other nonmedical persons.

In this dispute, lines are apt to be drawn according to professional identity. Psychiatrists, who are physicians, tend to claim that psychotherapy is a medical practice. Psychologists, who are not physicians, tend to claim that it is not a medical practice. These lines are not sharply drawn, however, since some psychiatrists advocate lay therapy. Also, many psychologists maintain that mental illness is like any other illness, even though this implies that it should be treated (or at least that treatment ought to be supervised) by a physician. Lines are drawn also according to the social function of the therapist. Physicians and psychologists who practice in institutional settings tend to use the medical model to describe and explain psychotherapy. Those who engage exclusively in private practice tend more to accept social and communicational (nonmedical) models.

Although they seem to be delineated by professional identity and social function, the arguments for and against the use of the medical model are usually theoretical and abstract, rather than sociological and economic.[5] Undoubtedly, views of some therapists about the medical nature of psychotherapy are influenced by these theoretical arguments. However, the division of convictions along professional and functional lines indicates that other than intellectual factors are at work. If this were not true, a more random distribution of convictions among psychiatrists and psychologists about the medical nature of psychotherapy would be expected.

Whether or not psychotherapy is a medical activity is not a fact to be discovered by scientific inquiry. It is a matter of a preference between conceptual models. One particular conceptual model may be preferred to others because it better explains or "fits" the relevant facts. A conceptual model, however, may also be selected because it promotes or avoids interfering with social interests and functions. These social factors may be the more important determinants of the medical or nonmedical definitions of psychotherapy.

. Theoretical arguments for the use of the medical model in psychotherapy are based, in one way or another, on the presumption that psychotherapy is a form of treatment for mental illness. These arguments, in their general form, have been considered in other chapters and will not be further discussed here. This chapter will discuss the manner in which the medical framework for conceptualizing psychotherapy facilitates certain social interests and functions and impedes others. To do this, the social functions of psychotherapy must be described.

There are three functions of the use of the medical model in psychotherapy. First, the use of medical rhetoric promotes the economic and social interests of a particular group—psychiatrists and others directly involved in the mental health movement. Second, the use of medical rhetoric helps to professionalize psychotherapy and thus to assimilate it into society. Third, the medical model helps to disguise the two primary social functions of psychotherapy, which, if their nature were openly recognized, would conflict, in different respects, with important features of the contemporary social fabric.

THE ECONOMIC FUNCTION OF THE MEDICAL MODEL IN PSYCHOTHERAPY

There are historical reasons for describing psychotherapy[6] with medical language. Freud, who was most responsible for developing and popularizing psychoanalytic psychotherapy, was a physician. However, as Freud himself said, this is neither here nor there.[7] The origin of modern psychotherapy in medicine is no more adequate grounds for claiming that it is a "genuinely" medical activity than the discovery of America by a sailor flying the Spanish flag is adequate grounds for claiming that continent to be "genuinely" Spanish.

In its beginnings in Europe, psychoanalysis was vigorously rejected by the medical profession.[8] In spite of this opposition it survived, due mostly to the efforts of Freud and his followers. Because Freud was a privately practicing therapist and a Jew, he remained outside of organized medicine. Consequently, in Europe, organized medicine did not gain control over the training and certification of therapists as it did in America. In the United States, psychoanalysis and psychotherapy were adopted primarily by psychiatrists who worked in asylums, hospitals and clinics.[9] As a result, psychotherapy developed in the context of organized medicine.

In 1937, the American Psychoanalytic Association broke with the International Psychoanalytic Association by asserting that psychoanalysis was a medical discipline that should be practiced by physicians only. In this claim, it was soon joined by the American Medical Association and the American Psychiatric Association. These organizations have lobbied for state legislation that defines psychotherapy as medical in nature and that prohibits its practice by nonphysicians, although these laws are usually ambiguous and unenforced.[10]

In general, the medical profession has favored the medical definition of psychotherapy, and the psychological profession —the main competitor for the psychotherapeutic franchise— has led attempts to redefine psychotherapy as a nonmedical practice. Each of these positions is obviously to their respective financial advantage. Both groups, however, have wavered in their convictions on this matter when it has been to their economic benefit to do so.

Following World War II, when the G.I. Bill provided funds for readjusting servicemen to civilian life, psychoanalytic institutes redefined training analysis as educational rather than therapeutic so that institute candidates could quality for aid under this Bill.[11] In a few years, the number of eligible candidates for the G.I. Bill dwindled. A new source of financial aid for analytic candidates was then sought in our income tax laws. However, until the Fall of 1966, psychiatrists could not claim the cost of training analysis as a tax deductible business expense because, according to the Bureau of Internal Revenue and the tax courts, training analysis was for the purpose of acquiring new skills rather than for improving existing skills. Analytic candidates could not claim their personal analysis as a deductible medical expense because it was required by training institutes as an integral part of training.

Faced with this dilemma, and with the need to find financial relief from the heavy expenditures of training analysis, psychoanalytic institutes attempted once again to redefine training analysis as medical treatment, so that it could be deducted as a medical expense. In 1966, however, the U.S. Court of Appeals reversed an earlier tax ruling and allowed the deduction of training analysis on the grounds that it could also be used to improve skills in a preexisting profession, namely general psychiatry.[12]

Commenting on this situation, Szasz stated:

> For income tax purposes, psychoanalysis is treated differently depending on the patient's occupation: it is deductible as a medical expense by the housewife; as a business expense by the internist; it may or may not be deductible as a medical expense by the psychiatrist who is not officially in training; and it is completely nondeductible by the analytic candidate. What sort of *medical treatment* is this? Certainly we would be hard put to think of any disease, other than that allegedly cured by analysis, the treatment of which is medical or nonmedical depending on the patient's occupational status.[13]

Psychologists also participate in financially expedient definitions of psychotherapy. Psychologists have advocated the use of a nonmedical model of illness so they could participate in new federally supported community mental health center programs. They have advocated conceptualizing psychotherapy in terms of learning theory. They have advocated constructing community mental health centers away from hospitals and medical centers, and they have advocated non-discrimination toward psychologists in assigning positions of responsibility in these programs.[14] Clinical psychologists, on the other hand, have attempted to define themselves as *health* professionals to be eligible to receive payment from medical insurance programs for psychotherapeutic treatment of "mental illness."[15]

Dr. Arthur Brayfield, the executive officer of the American Psychological Association, has commented on this inconsistency:

> . . . psychologists may reconceptualize the problem of mental health and make explicit their independent and unique role. This is the case when psychology focuses upon the developmental approach to *psychological fitness*, to *human effectiveness*, or to *social competence* in place of the medical model of illness and disease . . .
>
> Interestingly, however, this statement itself, when read in conjunction with the other recent APA "White Paper" on *The Psychologist in Voluntary Health Insurance*, illustrates our inconsistency with respect to our role as a health profession. The community mental health center paper espouses a nonmedical model and casts doubt on individual psychotherapy as a major approach; the insurance paper essentially accepts the medical model and the utility of one-to-one psychotherapy.[16]

This inconsistency demonstrates that an important function of the medical rhetoric in describing psychotherapy is social and economic rather than logical and scientific. The psychiatrist may deny that his argument for a medical definition of psychotherapy is economically motivated. He may argue the merits of his position entirely on the ground that mental illness is like any other illness and requires the technical expertise of the physician to be practiced competently. He may claim that the underlying motive for his argument is a concern for patient welfare rather than for self-enrichment.[17] Economic motives, however, are known to operate in human affairs, even among the most idealistic and dedicated professional groups. There is no reason dogmatically to exclude the possibility that they operate in the affairs of psychiatrists.

The medical model serves as a trademark that brings psychotherapy under the medical franchise to supervise, regulate, and control. This reduces competition from other merchants of this service and, accordingly, increases the demand for and the value of the psychiatrist's services. Although dispensing with the medical definition of genuinely medical diseases and treatments would be impossible, both psychiatrists and psychologists have made such a dismissal of "mental illness" and psychotherapy when it has been to their financial advantage.

THE FUNCTION OF THE MEDICAL MODEL
IN THE PROFESSIONALIZATION OF PSYCHOTHERAPY

Psychotherapy is a specialized activity requiring special knowledge and training. This is true whether described as a medical activity or as an activity similar to the priest's, the educator's, or the television repairman's. The psychotherapist is therefore a specialist. There are, presumably, standards by which his performance may be judged as adequate or inadequate, helpful or harmful, and properly represented or fraudulent.

One of the functions assumed by the modern state, as well as by certain nongovernmental agencies, is to establish standards of training, accreditation, and licencing for various social activities. With the guidance and supervision of the appropriate experts, these watchdog agencies regulate and control certain social activities to insure that they will be performed in the interests of the public, with skill and competence. These agencies regulate and supervise the quality of educational and training programs, they establish standards for certification and licencing, they establish guidelines for judging competence, and they establish rules that govern the responsibility of the specialist with respect to the property and persons he serves.

Psychotherapy may be classified as a personal service occupation. As such, the psychotherapist is regulated by governmental as well as professional groups. An important step in the professional regulation of psychiatry occurred in 1844, when a group of mental hospital administrators formed the precursor to the American Psychiatric Association. The purpose of this association, like that of other professional associations, was: to facilitate communication among persons performing related social functions; to protect the social and economic interests of this group; to establish and administer standards of professional deportment, responsibility, and performance; and to foster conditions conducive to fulfilling these standards and responsibilities. This group was well established when psychoanalysis was introduced into the United States by doctors who had travelled abroad to study with Freud. Consequently, psychotherapy, as a helping service, not only was defined, described and explained by means of the medical model, but also was institutionalized within the framework of organized medicine.

The jurisdiction of medicine over psychoanalysis was solidified and extended by successful lobbying for legislation that defined psychotherapy as a medical activity and forbad its practice by nonphysicians. Thus, organized medicine satisfied the requirement that new social activities (or, more properly in this case, new forms of old social activities) be regulated and controlled for the benefit of the consumer. If this had not been done by medicine, it would have likely been done by some other professional or governmental group. It is entirely conceivable for psychotherapy to be regulated by a group of nonphysicians. However, historical precedents are difficult to reverse, as is demonstrated by the frustrated attempts of modern psychologists to share with psychiatrists regulatory jurisdiction over the practice of psychotherapy. However important the language of medicine for defining psychotherapy as a medical activity, the social and legal jurisdiction of medicine over psychotherapy is far more important.

There is an ironic aspect of the professionalization of psychotherapy within medicine. One of the functions of the medicalization of psychotherapy is to regulate and control its practice. Psychiatrists, however, are unable to agree on a definition of psychotherapy. After four years of deliberation, a committee of the American Psychoanalytic Association found it impossible to find a definition of psychoanalysis that would be acceptable to a sufficiently large group of Association members. The committee also reported a strong resistance to any attempt to evaluate the results of psychotherapy. The same confusion and uncertainty reigns with respect to nonanalytic psychotherapy.

How can a professional group regulate an activity it is unable to define and unwilling to evaluate? The answer, obviously, is that it cannot. There are no acceptable standards of psychotherapeutic performance as there are, for example, standards of adequate surgical performance. This is due in part to psychotherapy's being conducted in private. Medical patients are sometimes able to judge for themselves whether the possibility of malpractice exists, and this judgment may be measured against prevailing community standards of medical treatment. But there are so many varieties of psychotherapeutic theory and technique that therapists themselves have no established standards by which to judge the effectiveness or harmfulness of their activities.

The only standards that psychiatric groups have attempted to establish for psychotherapy are the credentials of those who practice it. So long as the therapist is a physician, preferably with psychiatric training, he is considered by organized medicine to be eligible to practice psychotherapy. As a result psychotherapy is not regulated.

Even the ordinary canons of medical ethics do not apply

in psychiatry. Except in an emergency, no physician would attempt to treat a person without his consent. Psychiatrists, however, do "treat" involuntary patients. A psychotherapist may do anything within the law and be immune from the charge that he is incompetent, negligent, or malicious. All he need do is claim that his activities are for his patient's benefit. He may sit silently, mumble inanities, give advice, moralize, dispense drugs, issue threats, administer electric shocks, or give his patients affection and support. Almost anything that takes place between a psychiatrist and his patient has been labelled as psychotherapy, including a casual weekly greeting to an otherwise totally ignored hospital inmate.

Aside from the insistence that a psychiatrist must be a physician, or be under the supervision of a physician, the regulation of psychotherapy by medicine is illusory. It is designed primarily to entrench the practice of psychotherapy in medicine rather than to regulate training and practice according to specifiable, professional standards of competence.

THE MEDICAL MODEL AS A DISGUISE
FOR THE SOCIAL FUNCTIONS OF PSYCHOTHERAPY

Generally speaking, psychotherapy is considered to be like other medical treatments, a procedure for the alleviation of human suffering and the correction of human disability. Just as the man with a crippled leg or heart may suffer and be unable to fulfill his social and economic responsibilities, so, it is thought, a man with a "crippled" mind suffers, is unable to meet his responsibilities and is unable to establish satisfactory human relationships. Just as the task of the medical physician is to relieve suffering and to repair the hurt leg or the injured heart, so, it is thought, the function of the psychotherapist is to repair the disabled mind and personality, to restore effective psychological functioning, and to help adapt the personality to its social environment. The two types of activity, medical and psychotherapeutic, are considered to have the same general social significance.

Health and disease, whatever else they may be, express social and ethical standards of bodily status, psychological experience, and social behavior. Mental illness is a deviation from social standards of behavior—in which case psychotherapy must be viewed in the socio-political context of institutionalized methods for dealing with social deviance—or mental illness represents a deviation from personal standards of happiness, well being or social effectiveness—in which case, psychotherapy must be viewed as an institutionalized method for providing personal consolation, guidance, or education. In either case, the vocabulary of health and illness, of diagnosis and healing, is narrow and misleading. It is narrow because it fails to convey the social significance and cultural complexity of psychotherapy and the problems with which it deals. It is misleading because it leads our minds to the paradigm of medicine for explanation and illumination, rather than to the paradigms of social control, socialization, education, and religious guidance.

The more we think of psychotherapy as a specialized medical procedure for treating "mental illness," the less we tend to think of it in any other way. At a minimum, therefore, the medical model distracts us from other, possibly more fruitful ways of viewing psychotherapy. Other models of psychotherapy, however may not be solely more fruitful; they may be distasteful. They may describe psychotherapy in terms that would make it socially unacceptable because it would then visibly conflict with certain social values and ideals. In this sense, the medical model of psychotherapy is not simply a distracting historical accident without continuing social significance. The advantage of disguising the functions of psychotherapy in the rhetoric of medicine serves a defensive purpose, to distract us from objectionable aspects of an otherwise useful practice.

Large and expanding varieties of psychotherapies are currently in vogue, and there are numerous ways to classify them. For the purposes of this discussion two general types of psychotherapy will be distinguished on the basis of the social power of the therapist—"ethnicizing psychotherapy"[18] and "educative psychotherapy." As their names imply, these two forms of therapy are related to the functions of socialization and social control on the one hand and education on the other. In addition to being distinguished by their social function and by the use of social power as a "therapeutic" instrument, they belong to different historical traditions of behavorial guidance. These forms of therapy will be described, as will the social functions they serve, their relationship to each other and the purpose served by the use of the medical model.

ETHNICIZING PSYCHOTHERAPY

Ethnicization may be defined as the molding and polarizing of behavior so that it conforms to prevailing cultural patterns. It is indoctrination or training for culturally specific traits, attitudes, and actions.[19]

Ethnicization requires the use of social power and influence. The paradigmatic ethnicizing situation is in the family where the power of the parents helps to shape the child into the kind of adult who can participate in the social dramas of the group.[20] The family may be construed as a mediator between the individual and the larger society. In the final analysis, the social power of the collective provides the rewards and punishments that are the inducements to conform to prevailing standards of social behavior.

While every psychotherapeutic encounter may promote ethnicization, this is the explicit purpose of one form of therapy. Its aims may be specified in terms of particular traits, attitudes, and actions to be adopted by the patient, and those aims correspond to prevalent patterns of the group or subgroup within which the patient and the therapist live and work. Often, these aims are formulated in abstract terms, for instance, as the integration of personality, adaptation, self-realization, or the fulfillment of potential. In this form of therapy, however, these terms may be instantiated with actions and attitudes that systematically include cultural virtues and exclude cultural vices.

Ethnicizing therapy may thus be employed to transform an individual's homosexual patterns into heterosexuality, to influence a criminal to be law-abiding, to encourage a truant student to attend school regularly, to persuade a frigid wife to be more receptive to her husband, and so on.

As do other activities that have the aim of socialization and ethnicization, this form of psychotherapy requires the use of social power or social influence by the therapist over the patient. What kind of social power and influence does the psychotherapist possess? To answer this question the socio-economic situations in which psychotherapy is conducted must be examined.

Ethnicizing Psychotherapy and Social Power

Broadly speaking, psychotherapy is conducted in three different social settings: (1) the total institution, in which the therapist is employed by the institution and the patient is an inmate of it—state mental hospitals, prisons, and the military services; (2) the bureaucratic setting, in which the therapist is employed by a public or private agency and the patient, under pressure or voluntarily, seeks his services—the public mental health clinic, public schools, and industry; (3) the entrepreneurial situation, in which the therapist practices privately for a fee and the patient, under pressure or voluntarily, seeks his services.[21]

Ethnicizing psychotherapy may be practiced in each of these settings. As a general rule, the power of the therapist over his patient is greatest in the institutional setting, relatively less in the bureaucratic setting, and least in the entrepreneurial setting. However, this generalization requires refinement.

In each of these psychotherapeutic settings, the patient may be more or less voluntary, or more or less coerced into the role of patient. Coercive power may be exercised at various social levels. It may be exercised by the state, by means of the commitment of the patient to a mental hospital; it may be exercised through social, legal, and economic pressures by an employer, a school, the courts, welfare agencies, the family, and so on, or it may be exercised by means of psychological pressures from the family or community. At each level, it is presumed that if the patient refuses to cooperate in therapy, or if he withdraws from it, he will be subjected to social penalties. The power of the therapist over his patient is therefore linked to the power of third parties: government agencies, the patient's employers, his school, his family and so on.

The psychotherapist has enormous power over the patient in a psychiatric hospital by virtue of being linked with the power structure of the hospital, which, in turn, is linked with the power of the local community establishment and with the state. The committed psychiatric patient may sense that this complex linkage has cooperated in bringing about his loss of freedom. Whether a hospital patient is voluntary or committed, the duration of his confinement will be determined by his therapist, by the hospital administrators and indirectly, by the community. In this sense, all hospital patients are involuntary in that they cannot terminate the therapeutic relationship when they wish. Finally, the hospital psychiatrist has the dictatorial power to determine the quality of the patient's institutional life: he determines the freedom of the patient's movement in the wards, on the grounds, and during leaves from the hospital; he determines recreational privileges; he decides who may visit the patient and how often, and he decides whether to prescribe powerful drugs, electro-shock therapy, and even lobotomy.[22]

The power of the hospital therapist over his relatively helpless patient constitutes the immediate social context in which psychotherapy is conducted. The patient's behavior in therapy, and in the hospital where he is carefully observed, is the basis for the therapist's decisions about his privileges and ultimate freedom. The patient who wishes to regain his freedom, or short of that at least to have as pleasant an institutional life as possible, must become sensitive to and respond to his therapist's desires. The social power of the hospital therapist is thus an important instrument in the resocialization of the psychiatric patient.

In the bureaucratic setting, the power of the therapist over the patient is more variable and subtle. The clinic therapist may exercise power over his patient by actively cooperating with any third parties who may have coerced the patient into the psychotherapeutic role. In such a case, the therapist, in effect has at least as much social power over the patient as have those parties, since he cues them as to whether or not they should use their power.

For example, a judge may give a person who has been accused of a sexual offense the "choice" of entering psycho-therapy or going to jail. The aim of therapy will be ex-plicitly to alter his sexual attitudes and behavior; and the "inducement" to this change is, in part, the threat of con-finement in jail if the therapist cannot reassure the court that the patient is no longer a threat to the community. In effect, the therapist has the power, by saying the word to the judge, to imprison his patient.

Other examples of the collaboration of the therapist with powerful third parties are cases in which a business, school, or military service refers a patient to a psychiatrist whom they employ and pay. Perhaps the patient does not seem to be getting along well with his co-workers or co-students; or perhaps the employer believes that the patient is not working at his top efficiency. The aim of therapy will be to influence the patient to get along better with others or to improve the effectiveness of his work. The patient knows that the ther-apist, by communicating with the employer, may cause him to be fired, expelled, or discharged. This represents a rather powerful inducement to the patient to respond to the therapist's influence.

The therapist may not actively cooperate with the coercive third parties, but may simply inform them as to whether or not the patient is continuing in therapy. This may occur, for instance, if the therapist is the employee of a public clinic rather than the direct employee of the third party. With this lesser information, the third party takes as the cue for action the continuation or noncontinuation of the patient in therapy; the former is taken as an index of the cooperation of the patient; the latter is taken as an index of his recalcitrance, which may justify the use of punitive social power. In any case, the therapist is perceived as a figure who may be instrumental in determining the course of the patient's social life; and to impress the therapist favorably, the patient is likely either to become more receptive to the therapist's influence or to attempt to deceive him into thinking that he is.

The therapist may also exercise power over his patient by threatening him with commitment if he does not conform to the therapist's wishes. Or, the therapist may simply refuse to renounce psychiatric committment. This refusal constitutes an implied threat to the patient, since it is common knowledge that psychiatrists commit "mentally ill" persons and administer institutions in which such persons are confined. Unless the therapist renounces commitment, therapy will be conducted in circumstances in which the patient will be unsure whether he will be penalized for his behavior; this uncertainty may serve to reinforce the influence of the therapist.

Even if the clinic therapist refuses to communicate with a third party, and even if he renounces psychiatric commitment as a possibility, he cannot insure the patient complete confidentiality; and this lack of assurance may serve as a constraint on the patient. In the setting of the public clinic, the therapist is paid by and accountable to government. The patient's visits to the clinic become a matter of public record which, while not casually revealed to anyone, may be made available to governmental or private interests upon proper application. The patient at a public clinic is thus vulnerable to the possibility of social defacement in the future should the fact become known that he received psychiatric therapy. Perhaps he will not get a job because of it, or he may fail to obtain security clearance from the government, or he may suffer from some other social disadvantage. This comprises the context in which therapy is conducted and may influence the patient in varying degrees.

In the private therapeutic situation, the therapist may also have considerable social power over his patient. The private therapist, like his colleague in the clinic, may see patients who come to him under pressure from third parties. He may actively cooperate with these parties and attempt to influence the patient in the direction of their interests. Or, he may keep them informed about whether or not the patient continues in therapy. This is particularly hard to avoid if these third parties are paying the bill. The private therapist may also threaten his patient with psychiatric commitment as a penalty for certain behavior, or he may refuse to renounce the possibility of such an action. Unlike the clinic therapist, however, the private therapist may, if he wishes, assure the patient that confidentiality will be totally respected.

The therapist may exercise another kind of power over his patient—whether the patient be voluntary or coerced and whether therapy be in the institutional, the bureaucratic or the entrepreneurial setting. This power derives from the most basic elements of the relationship between the individual and society.

This power of the therapist is derived from the *authority of the group* that sanctions him as a healer, as a wise man of science, as an expert in human affairs, and as a man of Good, if not of God. This power of the therapist over his patient is thus derived from the same source as the power of parents over their children. It is universally employed to transmit the form and contents of culture from the group to the individual. The susceptibility of the adult individual to the influence of this power has its origins in his helplessness as a child. It is reinforced by a long period of conditioning in which the continued use and threat of social power promotes a continued deference to social authority. It predisposes him to a continued responsiveness to the social directive systems, which cue perception, feeling, thought, and action throughout adult life.

The tendency of the individual to defer to figures of authority and to cultural directive systems is the Oedipus complex in its larger social dimensions.[23] More narrowly conceived, the Oedipus complex portrays this social theme as a family drama in which the power and authority of the father (as cultural representative) are used to induce the child to renounce an infantile-erotic (physical) relationship with his mother in favor of more distant, symbolic modes of relating.

The Oedipal mystique is brought into play in ethnicizing psychotherapy. The therapist is a sanctioned representative of supreme social authority, regaled in the particular image of what is Right, Good, and effective in a particular culture. The patient is regarded as a poorly ethnicized child who is described in the particular cultural rhetoric for labelling deviance and ineptitude. The powers of the tribe, the priest, the father, and the therapist derive from the same social repository and are brought to bear on the individual, the penitent, the child, and the patient to influence them to perceive, feel, think, and act in a socially desirable manner. Social power, charisma, the Oedipus complex, and transference are all different manifestations of the same basic social dynamic. People tend to believe that which is to their best interests. The social power and the "power mystique" of the therapist influence the patient into believing that it is in his best interests to think and act in the manner suggested by the therapist.

This form of power over his patient permits the ethnicizing therapist to set conditions for the patient's conduct outside of therapy. For instance, the therapist may disapprove of or explicitly require that his patient desist from crime, suicide, homosexuality, sexual promiscuity, divorce, and other acts the therapist believes to be contrary to the patient's or to society's best interests.[24] This not only has the immediate effect of influencing the patient to avoid "immoral" and "deviant" behavior, but it consecrates the authority of the therapist so that he may more effectively influence the patient in other ways.

The therapist may also control and direct his patient by formulating the goals of therapy for him. Representative of the aims of ethnicizing therapy are those given by Karl Menninger: improved relationships with one's parents; the development of attitudes and actions appropriate to one's gender; the fostering of a "mature" heterosexual partnership, preferably in marriage; moderation in play; sportsmanship and social participation; increased productivity, creativity and satisfaction; and the obliteration or diminution of feelings of covetousness and power-seeking.[25] One can readily see that the goals of ethnicization, schooling, and ethnicizing psychotherapy are similar.

Few writers mention the central role played by social power in ethnicizing psychotherapy. Even the conditioning therapists, who emphasize the importance of rewards and punishments in learning, have failed to appreciate the intense rewards and punishments provided by the use of social power. However, social power is a fact of life, and its role in ethnicizing psychotherapy is of the highest importance. It intertwines the therapist into every level of the social fabric. Institutional psychotherapy is conducted with the explicit sanction of state power. The ethnicizing therapist in the bureaucratic or private setting may link himself with the state, the military, the world of commerce, the local community, and the family to influence and alter the behavior of his patient. Finally, the socially sanctioned authority of the therapist combines with the general susceptibility of individuals to comply with whatever is defined as socially approved, Right, and Good to form the most forceful influence on the patient's thoughts, feelings, and conduct. Indeed, to influence an individual, one need know little about him, or even about therapeutic technique, if only one has social power over him.

The Social Function of Ethnicizing Psychotherapy

In primitive societies the functions of socialization and social control were performed primarily by the extended family, the kin-group, and the community. The priest-magician was employed only in extreme and unusual cases. With the decline in community and the extended family, specialists in socialization and social control supplement the family in these functions. In the medieval world, one of the main functions of the Church was to provide a system of "spiritual" direction. It promoted the development of conscience—the internalized representative of social authority and values. It supplied casuists to apply the principles of conscience to individual problems of conduct. And it developed special techniques for reforming deviant and perplexed consciences (persons)—the so-called *Cura Animarum*.

With the secularization of culture, the state has taken over many functions related to socialization and social control. Schools, for example, are relatively recent in Western history and are designed to supplement the family in the preparation of the young for adult social life. We do not tend to think of schools as instruments of the state designed to socialize the young, but that is precisely what they are. Police agencies, courts, and penal institutions are also specialized instruments of the state designed to detect, apprehend, judge, and correct deviant persons.

Ethnicizing psychotherapy is an elaborately developed supplement to our educational and penal institutions. It may be used to correct and alter the perceptions, feelings, thoughts, and behavior of persons who are judged to deviate from prevailing standards of social conduct. It may be used not only with criminals, but also with persons who have violated our informal standards of social decorum, propriety, and etiquette.[26] It may be used to correct persons who do not express themselves in conformity with prevalent linguistic forms—persons who are labelled as "schizophrenics"—with persons who do not display the correct mood or pace of activity— "depressives" and "manics"—with persons who complain about their bodies without medical basis—"hysterics" and "hypochondriacs"—with persons who fear ordinary objects or places they are expected to encounter without fear—"phobics"

—with persons who antagonize, offend or otherwise draw social criticism for their behavior—"character disorders"—and so on. Ethnicizing psychotherapy may be used to correct all the forms of social deviance to which the name "mental illness" is assigned.

Ethnicizing therapy may also be used to provide an intense, personalized supplementary ethnicizing experience for persons who judge themselves to be confused, unhappy, and inadequately prepared to engage in the complex social acts required in modern life. These persons are usually not labelled mentally ill (although they are eligible) because they are able to function adequately from the point of view of others, even though they are unhappy or dissatisfied with their own performance and experiences. Such persons may consult a psychiatrist voluntarily to deal with their personal problems.

The ethnicizing psychotherapist is thus a functional equivalent of and replacement for the traditional extended family structure, the casuist, and the spiritual guide. He is a supplement to the modern educator and penologist. His effectiveness is based upon his actual social power, which in turn is derived from his alliance with the state, business and industry, community organizations, and the family. His effectiveness is also based upon his social status as a wise man and healer and upon the susceptibility of individuals to the directives of sanctioned social authority. Finally, the effectiveness of the ethnicizing psychotherapist is based upon his skill in using these advantages to control and modify the thoughts, feelings, and behavior of his patients.

The Function of the Medical Disguise of Ethnicizing Psychotherapy

The medical model of psychotherapy serves the same function as the medical model of the psychiatric hospital. It serves to shield us from embarrassing facts about our social system that we otherwise would have to face. It shields us from the coercive and manipulative techniques we use to reform and correct certain deviant and unhappy individuals by disguising these techniques as medical treatment.

Consider that if so-called mental illness is, as the mental hygiene movement claims, one of the most important public "health" problems today, we must admit that there are many more deviant persons in our society than we have publicly acknowledged, and there are many more unhappy people than we have led ourselves and the world to believe.

It is one thing to say that mental illness is a major health problem as are heart disease and stroke: this enjoins us to subsidize medical research into the causes of these problems and to search for specialized medical antidotes or treatments without, however, having to examine and reevaluate the basic fibers of our social fabric.

It is quite another thing to say that the problem of mental illness reflects the inadequacy of the family to socialize the young; the ineffectiveness of the school to prepare individuals for the complexities of adult life; the failure of both traditional morality and present behavioral directive sytems; the irrevelance of the Christian Church to problems of conduct; the difficulty of creating and sustaining meaning in a complex, secular, industrial society; and our basic dissatisfaction with the Rule of Law as a method for dealing with social deviance. To describe the significance of the "problem of mental illness" in this way is to criticize the very foundations and fabric of our society.

The medical model of psychotherapy shields us from the full impact of and, therefore, from a full understanding of the relationship between social structure and the behavior that we label as mental illness. It disguises our collective shame about the failures of our social institutions that produce, or at least fail adequately to deal with, the deviance, inadequacy, and personal troubles that we label as mental illness. How consoling it is to disguise our social failures as diseases: as infirmities of the mind that arise independently from moral considerations or social arrangements. And how reassuring it is to label as "medical treatment" our attempts to deal with these problems.

Without a medical disguise, our attempts to deal with these problems would be objectionable because these attempts are incompatible with certain public values. We are sensitive to the dangers of tyranny and the loss of human dignity. We publicly value the principle of Rule of Law, according to which only persons who violate specific laws are punished, and then only after due process. According to the First Amendment to the Constitution, we are opposed to the establishment of a state religion, which means, in part, that we are opposed to the use of state power to enforce any particular religious morality. We are also dedicated to the principles of the freedom, dignity, and responsibility of the individual. We oppose the alignment of giant powers against him (a principle expressed in the Fifth Amendment); we renounce the use of brainwashing and coercion to maintain social order; and we disdain treating adults as children.

If we view ethnicizing psychotherapy in social rather than in medical terms, it is clear that it *systematically violates each of these social values*. In the setting of the public mental hospital, psychotherapy is a state function. The patient has been confined by the state, by means of psychiatric commitment, in spite of the fact that he has violated no specific law. His confinement is based upon his deviation from standards that are codified in mental health manuals and that are agreed to and enforced by the state. The psychotherapist in a public mental hospital is a state employee who uses state power to influence his patients to conform to the paralegal mental health rules of psychiatrists. These mental health rules largely coincide with Judeo-Christian values and conventions. In this sense, psychiatry functions as an instrument of the state to enforce a secularized religious morality, the First Amendment notwithstanding.

In the clinic and private setting, the ethnicizing psychotherapist may mobilize the power of the state, of business and industry and of other community interests to influence and control his patient. When the power of the collective is used by other countries to influence the thoughts and actions of individuals, we are quick to label it as brainwashing and social coercion.[27] In this country, these processes are disguised as medical treatment. The ethnicizing psychotherapist may also treat his patients as nonresponsible, inadequate children who are expected to defer to the authority and wisdom of the therapist as if he were a parent. Indeed, in one form of psychotherapy the therapist explicitly plays a parental role to influence the thoughts, feelings, and actions of his patients.[28]

While the medical model may serve the purpose of enhancing our cultural self-image, we pay a great price for this consolation. It leads us to misname and misconstrue crucial human problems and our attempted solutions for them.[29] It persuades us that the problems are medical rather than social, economic, political, and religious and that the solutions are best left to the doctors, who with time and money enough, will find the cure for this "disease" as they have for so many others in recent years. The medical mask of psychotherapy thus serves an ideological function, since it deflects our attention from a critical evaluation of contemporary socialization, educational, and behavioral guidance practices by disguising our handling of their most blatant failures.

EDUCATIVE PSYCHOTHERAPY

A nonmedical account of ethnicizing psychotherapy is morally and politically repugnant because it exposes the use of social power to alter an individual's thoughts, feelings, and actions. There is another form of therapy, which will be called educative therapy (but which is also known as analytic, autonomous, and insight therapy), that is equally repugnant when viewed nonmedically, but for different reasons.

There has been a greater willingness for us to view psychotherapy as performing an educational function than to view it as performing the functions of ethnicization and social control. The reasons for this are obvious. Ethnicization is a function of the family, and social control is a function of the state. To view psychotherapy in terms of these functions is to view the therapist as a parent or a thought policeman and to view the patient as a child or a deviant person. Both of these paired perceptions conflict with our expressed cultural aspirations and values to treat adults as adults and to treat as deviants only those persons who have violated the law.

The educative model, however, is more dignified and more congenial to our social values. This model permits us to view the therapist as a teacher and the patient as a student, no different than a mature person enrolled in an adult education course. According to the educational model, the therapeutic transaction consists of a relatively harmless exchange of information. The patient speaks freely of his history, thoughts, dreams, and activities, and the therapist reveals to him hidden aspects of self. The insight that he gains will enable the patient to be a whole person, better integrated, more able to actualize his potential, and more able to participate creatively in social relationships. Because education is a nationally shared goal, unobjectionable on any count, many therapists who do not employ the medical model for psychotherapy select one or another variety of an educational model —learning theory, analysis, insight or schooling.

A comparison of educative psychotherapy to learning or schooling does not, however, completely clarify its social functions. This is because one function of schooling is, in fact, ethnicization—molding character in culturally defined directions.[30] Just as the ethnicizing therapist uses social power to influence his patients, and as the experimental psychologist conditions his laboratory animal or human subjects with rewards and punishments, the teacher uses social power to facilitate the student's learning. The school teacher is an agent of the state, the community, or the family, and uses

the power of these groups to punish, deface, expel, or de-
certify a student who does not respond to the "educational
message."

Indeed, the word "education" is often used as a euphemism
for ethnicization and social control. We speak of reeducating
criminals, juvenile delinquents, the mentally ill, narcotic ad-
dicts, captured enemy soldiers, and conquered countries and
villages. The term "education" has been turned to ideological
uses, to disguise the differences between ethnicization, brainwashing, rehabilitation, personal influence, social control, and
ordinary academic education.

The difference between ethnicization and education turns
on the pivot of social power.[31] Ethnicization involves the use
of social power to influence thought and conduct in socially
approved directions. Education involves the *analysis* of social
power, among other subjects, to understand its influence on
the lives of individuals and social groups.

Educative Psychotherapy and Social Power

In contrast to the ethnicizing therapist, the educative therapist does not attempt to mold his patient's behavior to *specific* legal, moral, and ethnic standards. He therefore has no
need to exercise social power over his patient. In the history
of psychotherapy, the relaxation of the therapist's power
over his patient began with Freud's scientific Weltanschau-
ung: with his desire primarily to understand his patients and
secondarily to help them.[32] This disavowal of power over
patients paved the way for psychoanalysis as a therapeutic
tool.[33]

The disavowal of attempts to control and mold the patient's behavior in specific cultural directions has several
practical implications for the conduct of therapy.[34] It implies
that the therapist must not ally himself with state, community, or familial interests. He must not communicate
with, collaborate with, or accept payment from anyone but
the patient. A corollary of this principle is that confidentiality

must be completely respected. The therapist must not communicate about the patient with anyone but the patient himself, regardless of whether the patient wants him to. The educative psychotherapist must also renounce the use of psychiatric commitment under any circumstances. Finally, the goals of therapy, as they involve specific activities, such as marriage, divorce, career, and social relationships, must be determined by the patient rather than by the therapist. The therapist must be concerned only with analyzing, and not dictating, his patient's life goals and methods for achieving them.[35]

There are technical as well as moral reasons for not intervening in the extratherapeutic life of the patient, either to control him or to help him. The moral reasons involve the values of self-determination and self-responsibility and the renunciation of social power over others. The technical reasons involve the freedom of communication in therapy. Social factors, as well as the desire to convey information, influence the nature of interpersonal communications. If the therapist uses his social power either to the patient's advantage or to his disadvantage, the patient will attempt to influence him in order to avoid punishment or to gain rewards. As a result, the free communication of information will be inhibited insofar as it might influence the therapist unfavorably.

Complete honesty and frankness in therapy therefore require complete assurance on the part of the patient that the therapist will not attempt to influence the course of his life outside of therapy. This means that the patient may choose to be deviant or immoral (including performing acts that may be labelled "mentally ill," such as attempted suicide) without being scolded, lectured, given drugs, committed, or otherwise manipulated by the therapist. Other persons or groups may punish or help the patient. The therapist's task is to understand him.

The varieties of psychotherapy must thus be distinguished on the basis of the social power of the therapist. In ethnicizing psychotherapies, the therapist employs social power to influence the patient to conform his thoughts, feelings, and conduct to social norms. In educative psychotherapy, the therapist avoids the use of social power so that he may better understand his patient and help him to understand and control himself.

The Social Function of Educative Psychotherapy

The educative psychotherapist functions not as an ethnicizer, reformer, or social controller, but as an educator. What kind of an education does the therapist provide for his patient? How is this education helpful in solving problems of living? What is the function of this education in sociological, rather than in psychodynamic, terms? Finally, why is this form of education so socially objectionable that it must be disguised with the medical (and other) model? To answer these questions it is necessary to understand how educative therapy works. To do this, certain psychoanalytic terms and concepts must be translated into ordinary language. In particular, the concepts of personal history, repression, the Oedipus complex, and the analysis of transference will be discussed.

Most psychotherapists help to educate their patients by describing and analyzing their thoughts, feelings, actions, and social relationships. However, the educative therapist's attention is not directed exclusively to his patient's current life situation. He also inquires into the history of his patient— into the patterns of child-rearing that form the determinants (precedents) for his current behavior. This is one of the most important differences between educative psychotherapy and other forms of therapy. Without an historical inquiry, the primary aims of educative psychotherapy cannot be realized.

Central to this historical inquiry is an analysis of the patient's relationship with his parents. This analysis brings several important issues into focus. It clarifies the complex relationship between the individual and society—between personality and culture. It brings into focus the relationship between repression, inhibition, and the process of ethnicization. It uncovers the relationship between ethnicization and social authority. Finally, it brings each of these issues into explicit relationship with the problems of the adult's conduct.

Since parents are the primary agents of the socialization and ethnicization of the young, the earliest and most formative impact of culture on the child's personality may be discovered in his relationships with his parents. These early learning experiences are important precedents that guide the individual's later conduct. One of the functions of inquiry is to enable the patient to learn about these early parental and cultural influences on his personal development and present conduct. In this sense, the therapist's task is not to transmit specific cultural values, but to make explicit the cultural values that have already been transmitted.

While recounting his early experiences, the patient learns how he has been conditioned to respond habitually and automatically to social cues. He learns not only how he has been cued by social authority and social context to perceive, think, feel, and behave in certain ways, but also how he has been cued to avoid perceiving, thinking, feeling, and behaving in certain ways. By becoming aware of these aspects of his biography, the patient learns about his "unconscious" and about the process of repression.

One function of repression is to control the "animal" tendencies of the individual, particularly his tendencies to respond to the impulses of nature in his pursuit of food and sex. This control is accomplished by inhibiting the thought and acting out of these impulses and by transforming them into socially acceptable and culturally specific forms. This is achieved primarily by a complicated process of conditioning and imitative adaptation in which the child is rewarded or punished according to the manner in which he displays socially acceptable behavior and avoids socially unacceptable behavior. By learning to avoid certain kinds of actions, the consciousness of these actions is repressed. Thus, the power of the parents to control and inhibit behavior by means of reward and punishment results also in repression—in thought-control. In the course of becoming inhibited and repressed, man becomes civilized; he becomes increasingly removed from the context of nature while refining his "higher" (more abstract) consciousness.[36] While this form of repression and inhibition is a necessary condition for civilization, it removes man from—indeed, sets him against—aspects of his own nature. This generates the conflict that, at the psychological level, is represented as the tension between the "id" (instinctual impulses) and the "super-ego" (social values). At the social level, this conflict is represented by the tension between the individual and society.[37] This tension is one source of personal trouble for the individual, especially in a society that is both puritanical and deregulated.[38]

A second aspect of repression and the unconscious is that we learn social rules and social games without being aware that we have learned them. A portion of the super-ego and of the ego are unconscious. The main reason for this is that conditioning is a simpler, more efficient form of learning than is conscious self-mastery. It would be inexpedient, even impossible to make the child aware of all the rules, attitudes, and values that he is expected to adopt or avoid. Indeed, the parents themselves are not aware of most of them.

This form of conditioned ethnicization works well in simple, coherent, and authoritarian societies. In our complex, incoherent, and open society, however, there is a disadvantage to this form of out-of-awareness (unconscious) learning that directly bears on the social and psychological problems of the adult. As societies become increasingly complex and heterogenous, the child is conditioned to learn contradictory thoughts, feelings, and actions. This predisposes him to psychological dissonance and conflict. Also, with an increased pace of social change, early training becomes increasingly irrelevant to the requirements of adult performance. It becomes increasingly difficult to train a child for all possible roles and social contingencies in adult life. Also, values, standards and social arrangements change from generation to generation so that parents become increasingly more inefficient as ethnicizers of the next generation. The behavioral rigidities learned in childhood may thus handicap the adult in his attempts to adjust to a changing social environment and to solve complex problems of conduct. The psychological and moral problems of the adult must thus be understood in the context of this early learning.

To learn to do something well is to learn not to do that thing poorly. Socialization and ethnicizing may thus be interpreted, in part, as processes of programmatic inhibition and repression. To learn something automatically or unconsciously is also to surrender the possibity of intelligently and flexibly modifying it to suit present purposes. Socialization and ethnicization may thus also be interpreted as learning behavioral rigidity and ineptness. The power of the parents (and of society) over the helpless child, which is the psychological "force" behind socialization and ethnicization, is thus also the "force" behind repression, inhibition, compulsion, and avoidance. This should not be surprising. At the political level, it is obvious that social power is used to inhibit men's actions, to control their minds and to specify their obligations. So it is in the family with the child. The power of the parents over the helpless child is analogous to the power of States, Kings and Gods. The susceptibility of the individual to the influence of authoritative persons and social conventions[39] is thus linked to his repressions, to his inhibitions, to his behavioral rigidities, and therefore, to his ineptness in solving for himself the complex problems of social life.

This relationship between ethnicization, repression, and social power is depicted allegorically in the psychoanalytic Oedipal mythology. According to psychoanalytic theory, the child develops a sexual longing for his mother from which he is dissuaded by his closest and most powerful rival, his father. As a result of this rivalry, the child develops a deep hostility toward the father. However, the power of the father is too threatening to the relatively helpless child. In self-defense, the child surrenders: he renounces his instinctual battle for the mother and instead joins forces with his enemy. He identifies with the father and strives to be like him in every way except his privileged sexual access to the mother. In psychoanalytic terms, this surrender is engineered by the development of the super-ego in reaction against the id, and by the repression and inhibition of instinctual (id) drives. The super-ego contains not only the ideals, prescriptions, and prohibitions of social conduct, but also "Religion, morality, and a social sense—the chief elements in the higher side of man."[40]

Broadly interpreted, the Oedipal mythology is the saga of socialization.[41] The child's desire for his mother (and father) is not a desire for a genital sexual relationship; it is a desire for the polymorphous sensual pleasures that the child derives from the satisfaction of his physical needs. The hostility towards the father (and mother) is not based on his (her) status as a sexual rival; it is based on the father's (and mother's) role as a socializer. The parents are figures of authority who insist that, at a certain age, the child abandon his impulsive spontaneity and physical intimacy in favor of the complicated systems of distant, symbolic behavior characteristic of the adult. The child is angry at his parents because he is being expelled from paradise into a world of sin and virtue where he must practice self-denial and self-control and suffer judgments and punishments.[42]

The passing of the Oedipus complex represents the full panorama of socialization and ethnicization. It marks the psychological "rite of passage" of the unformed child into the social group. It also involves learning repression and inhibition, automatic conditioning to social directive systems, and developing an abiding respect for parental and social authority. In a complex, rapidly changing social environment, these features of socialization make it difficult for the adult flexibly and intelligently to solve complicated and novel personal problems. They deprive the individual of self-knowledge, of a varied and flexible behavioral "repertoire," of self-reliance and of the capacity intelligently to match means to ends. They predispose him to personal and social "stupidity," to rigid and repetitive patterns of conduct, and to an obedient compliance with the contradictory directives of social authority.[43]

We are now in a position to understand the "therapeutic" functions of educative psychotherapy. An education in personal biography teaches the individual how he is shaped by the society in which he lives. The analysis of personal biography leads to the discovery of the values, attitudes, and behavioral predispositions which unconsciously have been learned or repressed. This, in turn, is linked to an analysis of the Oedipus complex—to an analysis of the influence of parental and social authority on the development of adult conduct. This issue becomes alive in therapy in the form of the transference. The transference represents the patient's persisting tendency to generalize from past experience.[44] It represents his tendency to superimpose his childhood experiences onto the therapeutic situation. The patient tends to adopt attitudes towards the therapist that reflect the precedents established during his relationship with his parents during childhood. The most important component of this early relationship was a respect for parental authority. During the transference, therefore, the patient invests the therapist with the crown and sceptre of parental authority even though the therapist has renounced the use of social power over the patient. (This is why it is so important for the educative therapist to do this.)

The analysis of the transference is therefore a simultaneous analysis of the childhood precedents of adult behavior, of repressions, inhibitions, and the psychological defenses that fortify them, of the influence of parental authority on the patient's thought and behavior, and of the patient's persisting tendency to defer to social authority and social power for guiding his conduct.

By becoming more aware of the social rules and games he blindly learned during childhood, the patient is in a better position to master his social performance. By becoming aware of what he has learned to avoid thinking and doing, the patient may expand his self-consciousness and his behavioral repertoire. By becoming more aware of the influence of parental and social authority on his thoughts and actions, the patient is better able to master his own conduct and increase his self-reliance; he will be able to acquire the skills for using his own critical intelligence to solve the problems of his life. Educative psychotherapy thus prepares the individual to solve the moral conflicts that result from inadequate socialization and from living in a complex, incoherent social environment. It prepares him for the complicated tasks of living in the modern world by increasing the flexibility of his conduct, by developing his psychosocial perceptiveness, and by fostering his capacity to determine his own future with intelligent choice.

From the historical point of view, educative psychotherapy is a radically novel kind of behavioral guidance system. It is a technique that developed in response to the need of the individual in a complex modern society to learn about and master his social environment by learning about and mastering his own conduct in it. Educative psychotherapy may thus be construed as a secular successor to traditional religion as a font of morality. However, it is not a morality of obedience to Father, Tribe, or God. It is a declaration of freedom from these figures as *ethical authorities*. It is a morality based on individual freedom, intelligence, and self-mastery rather than a morality based on the obedience to authority and to fixed formulae of obligation.

Educative psychotherapy is thus also radically different from ethnicizing psychotherapy in its historical origins, its techniques, its goals, and its values. It is designed to help the individual to master society, rather than to help society to master the individual. It advocates intelligence and self-control in matters of conduct, rather than automatic obedience to social authority. It functions to *analyze* the repressive influences of civilization, the tribe, the family, and special helpers rather than to use repressive and oppressive social power in the service of supplementary socialization and social control.

The Function of the Medical Disguise of Educative Psychotherapy

Educative psychotherapy is in conflict with fundamental forces of civilization in two ways. First, it rejects the coercive use of social authority and social power to mold *adults* to culture by repressing their consciousness and inhibiting their range of action. Second, by attempting to undo repression and automatic inhibition, educative psychotherapy reduces the alienation of human consciousness from the biological aspects of human nature. For these reasons, some of the most vigorous criticisms of educative psychotherapy (psychoanalysis) are that it tolerates, if not promotes, social deviance and sexual libertinism.

The charge is unfounded. Psychoanalysis, or educative psychotherapy, does not advocate social deviance, sexual libertinism, or the return to "natural" man. It recognizes that social authority and social power are necessary for socialization and social control. It also recognizes that for men to live together in harmony, they must control their spontaneous biological impulses. Educative psychotherapy is merely a program or technique for analyzing, and thus helping individuals to become aware of, the repressions and inhibitions that are ineluctably the result of socialization and ethnicization. The educative psychotherapist practices self-determination and self-control *as a therapeutic method*. This means that he neither condemns, praises, nor attempts to control the particular actions of his patients. The imputed danger of educative psychotherapist is to be found not in what the therapist might do, but in what his psychologically liberated patient might do. It is the nature of psychological freedom that the free man may do *anything*, including deviant and immoral acts, *without feeling guilt, shame, or anxiety.*

Educative psychotherapy is not opposed to society. Society is opposed to educative psychotherapy! This is because society is opposed to self-control and self-mastery; for the man who is in control of himself cannot always be controlled by social authority. Society is opposed to the elimination of guilt, shame, and anxiety; for these are the internal, psychological restraints that have replaced the tyranny of the community in the age of the individual. It is in the interest of society to produce a degree of repression; to encourage the inhibition of action by means of guilt, shame, and anxiety; and to foster the respect for and submission to social authority.

To say that it is in society's interest to control men's minds and actions is to say that it is in society's interest to prevent individuals from developing the social skills and knowledge necessary for them to be the masters of their own social performance. It is in society's interest to foster the kind of behavioral ineptness and deviance often labelled as "mental illness."

On the other hand, it is also in society's interest to rehabilitate its victims: the perplexed souls, the errant minds, and the confused actors. Educative psychotherapy is one method for doing this. If repression, inhibition, automatic learning, and an inflexible respect for authority foster personal ineptness and the varieties of behavior that we label as "mental illness," then it is not surprising that an activity that reverses these processes should constitute an antidote.

However, to a certain degree, the "needs" of society and the needs of its individual members conflict. To maintain a safe, predictable social order, society must repress and control individuals. To be in command of themselves, individuals must be informed and self-controlled. Like all antidotes, therefore, educative psychotherapy is dangerous. In attempting to combat the undesirable effects of socialization, it must weaken the hold of the social order on its individual members; it must combat unreflective obedience to social authority; it must combat repression and inhibition, and it must combat the emotional controls on moral action.

Because psychotherapy is useful to individuals even though potentially harmful to society, it is permitted to exist, but it is carefully controlled and disguised, like a dangerous secret. It has been given the code name of a medical technique for the treatment of mental illness. It has been reserved primarily for physicians to practice—a group which, because of its narrow training, is unlikely to see the social and historical significance of the instrument in its hands. Also, because of their strong medical training in the ethics of manipulative helpfulness, physicians are likely to transform the methods and aims of education into those of socialization and ethnicization. Indeed, instead of attempting to liberate their patients, psychiatrists have attempted to emulate physicians and surgeons, who manipulate their patients in the name of reducing their suffering and improving their adjustment to their environment.

Acting like a monstrous rational organism, society protects its interests by encouraging the conversion of a potentially subversive activity into one that promotes social conformity and tranquility. To the extent that educative psychotherapy is practiced, it is conducted in secret in the private consulting rooms of therapists, officially disguised as a medical activity. The subversive message that "mental health" means psychological freedom, self-control, and a socially critical intelligence is thus prevented by the medical model from spreading to the universities, to the popular literature, and to the man in the street.

CHAPTER SEVEN

━━━━━━━━━━━━━━━━━

Psychiatry and the Law

━━━━━

Language is a labyrinth of paths. You approach from one side and know your way about; you approach from another side and no longer know your way about.

—LUDWIG WITTGENSTEIN[1]

Our love of freedom requires that the criminal law protect the citizen accused of lawbreaking, otherwise we run the risk of the government overpowering the citizen. Our love of safety requires that the criminal law protect the community, otherwise we run the risk of individuals harming each other and destroying society. This is a dilemma every modern society must face.

—THOMAS S. SZSAZ[2]

━━━━━

The collaboration between psychiatry and law is based on the popular belief that they are fundamentally different—that law is a political institution concerned with codifying and regulating human conduct and that psychiatry is a value-free science concerned with mental health and disease. According to this view, the relationship of psychiatry to law is primarily consultative and advisory. The psychiatrist, like other medical experts, is thought to provide scientific information and opinion upon which legal decisions are based.

This belief is false. The basis for the collaboration between psychiatry and law is that they are fundamentally similar institutions that deal with the evaluation and control of human behavior. The law is an explicitly normative institution. Psychiatry is cryptonormative, since it disguises its evaluation and regulation of human conduct in the value-neutral rhetoric of science. In courts of law, serious decisions about human rights and freedoms are often based on vague, ambiguous laws. By cloaking itself in the rhetorical mantles of science and medicine, psychiatry may be used to lend the authority and certainty of science to these decisions, and it may be used to lend the benevolence of medicine to certain legal dispositions.

The paths of psychiatry and the law are joined at four distinct points: first, with laws, tests, and other legal rhetoric that use terms relevant to the mind or to mental illness; second, with the use of psychiatric "expert" witnesses in such legal procedures as the determination of responsibility and incompetence; third, with the use of psychiatric clinical and institutional facilities as instruments of observation, incarceration, and reform; and fourth, with the use of the mental health ideology as an ideal so that the aim of legal institutions is conceptualized, in part, in terms of guarding, promoting, and restoring the mental health of the community and of criminals.

The best known and most dramatic collaboration between psychiatry and the law occurs in the test of criminal responsibility, in which the defendant in a criminal trial attempts to establish the defense "Not guilty by reason of insanity." A close examination of the concept of criminal responsibility will demonstrate that, in these determinations, the psychiatrist serves not as a scientific expert, but as a linguistic arbiter and cryptic supplier of rules. It will also illustrate the social functions of psychiatry in law.

THE DETERMINATION OF CRIMINAL RESPONSIBILTY

The standard legal-psychiatric position on criminal responsibility stems from the principle of English Common Law that a person is accountable (punishable) for a crime only if he can be blamed for it and that blame shall not be attached under certain excusing circumstances—when a criminal act is committed without intent and when it is justifiable. Among the "nonpsychiatric" excusing conditions are accident and self-defense. The excusing condition associated with psychiatry is lack of intent due to insanity. If a person commits a criminal act while insane he is held not culpable for the crime and is excused from punishment. Definitions of insanity are given in particular legal tests, for instance, the test in M'Naghton's Case and the Durham Decision, which specify the criteria for determining the lack of intent due to insanity.

Most discussions of criminal responsibility give the impression that responsibility is a state of the individual that may be discovered by employing the proper methods of investigation.[3] It is argued that some individuals are responsible and that others are not. It is the function of the court, when responsibility is challenged, to determine which is which. The function of the psychiatrist is viewed as to provide expert testimony about the facts of an individual's responsibility or nonresponsibility. It is also a function of the psychiatrist as a behavioral scientist to advise jurists and legislators about the latest theories of responsibility so that legal procedures may be kept up to date.[4] According to this view, the determination of criminal responsibility is not an ethical and legal problem but a scientific one. The solution to this problem is to be found by using scientific techniques for discovering and identifying the state of responsibility.

However, the meaning of the term "criminal responsibility," like the meaning of the terms "deviance" and "mental illness," is to be found not only in the qualities of the individuals to whom it is ascribed, but also in the social position and power of those who use the term, the rules governing its use, the social contexts in which it is used, and the purposes for which it is employed.

To understand the scientific and social uses of the term "criminal responsibility" it will be helpful to analyze separately its component terms. This will reveal that, in the sense in which it is at all discoverable, nonresponsibility is more like discovering an infraction of the rules of a game than like discovering a deposit of ore or a cancer of the lung. Primarily required for the discovery of responsibility, therefore, is knowledge of the linguistic, social, and legal "games" in which the term is used, rather than scientific technique or knowledge about human nature.

To What Does the Word "Criminal" Refer?

The use of the word "criminal" cannot be separated from criminal law and legal procedure. In its cognitive use it may have two references. It may denote an acquired status ascribed to an individual by a legal procedure in which he has been judged guilty of violating a criminal statute. It may be used also to refer to a person who, it is presumed, would be judged criminal if he were brought to trial and if some excusing condition did not obtain. The first sense refers to a person who has actually been tried and found guilty. The second sense refers to a person who it is believed would be found guilty if he were tried. Strictly speaking, it would be more precise to call such a person "the accused" or "the suspect" rather than a criminal.

The Social Uses of the Word "Criminal"

These senses of the word "criminal" have a variety of uses (meanings). The first sense, "actually criminal," may be used to deface an individual socially—to induce others to shun him, to deny him employment, to vote against him, and so on. It may also be used to provoke an unauthorized person or group to serve punishment. The principal use for this sense of the term, however, is to enable the state legally to deprive an individual of his life, liberty, or property.

The second sense, "presumed criminal," may also be used to deface an individual socially—to induce others to treat him as if he really were a criminal and had been judged guilty in a courtroom trial. An illustration of this use of the term is Lee Harvey Oswald, who, although he did not live to be tried, is widely assumed to be guilty of the criminal act of murder—of presidential assassination. It may be used also to provoke some group to take the law into its own hands. It is important however that this sense of the term "criminal" cannot be used, under ordinary circumstances, legally to deprive an individual of life, liberty, or property.

To What Does the Word "Responsibility" Refer?

When a psychiatrist testifies about the responsibility or nonresponsibility of a defendant, it is assumed that the psychiatrist is referring to something.[5] To what is he referring?[6]

It is commonly assumed that the word "responsible" describes a person's mental condition—his capacity to form intent, to exercise moral judgment and to execute moral decisions. This assumption, however, raises serious epistemological questions as to whether other person's minds may be observed and described or whether their existence and contents may be logically inferred.[7] Without concerning ourselves with the intricacies of this problem,[8] let us say only that whatever we know of the mind of another is "based" on his public conduct—verbal and nonverbal. The terms "responsible" and "nonresponsible," then, concern a person's behavior.

To what aspects of a person's behavior do these words refer? They do not refer to his actions, to bits of conduct that may be discovered in addition to the facts about an alleged crime. We do not discover, for instance, that a man purchased a gun, drove across town, entered his mother-in-law's apartment, shot her dead, and was not responsible. If this were the case, witnesses and not scientific experts would be required to establish the responsibility of the defendant. A witness who observed a shooting would be required. The words "responsible" and "nonresponsible" do not refer to acts themselves but to the manner in which acts are carried out.

The term "responsible" is used to denote a person who displays the disposition to act responsibly. The term "nonresponsible" is used to denote a person who displays the disposition to act nonresponsibly. A person who *acts* responsibly is considered to be a responsible person, and the quality of responsibility is attributed to him. To understand the meaning of the term "responsibility" requires an inquiry into the rules governing the use of the word "responsibly."

Linguistic and Philosophic Factors that Influence the Use of the Word "Responsibly"

The word "responsibly" is used both in law and in ordinary language. How must a person behave for it to be properly said in ordinary language that he is behaving responsibly? This question is parallel to the question "How must a person behave for it to properly be said that he is behaving bravely?" These questions cannot be answered by technical, scientific methods. It is merely necessary to know certain ordinary facts about a person's behavior and to know the commonplace rules governing the uses of the words "bravely" and "responsibly." The behavioral scientist may give a detailed description of a man's actions, but he can know whether to describe them as brave or cowardly, as responsible or nonresponsible, only by referring to the ordinary, nontechnical conventions governing the uses of these words: certain actions are conventionally called "brave" and others are called "cowardly."

The word "responsibly" is used in ordinary language in three general ways: first, to indicate that a person is the author, cause, or occasion of something; second, to indicate that a person is accountable or answerable for his actions; third, to indicate that a person is properly discharging his obligations. The word thus lends itself easily to a socio-ethical use—to praise or to blame someone without indicating anything at all about that person. The rules governing the use of the term are thus as varied and complex as the rules and motives for blaming and praising people. These rules are not determined by scientists or linguists, but by ordinary persons in everyday circumstances.

One sense of the term "responsibility" in law refers to the authorship or cause of an act. Authorship (and therefore responsibility) is said to depend upon the capacity to form intent. An act formed with intent may be said to be freely chosen, and the author is therefore held responsible. An act performed without intent may be said to be unfree, caused, coerced, or accidental, and the author is judged to be not responsible.

The joining of the concepts of intent, free choice, and responsibility is based not on facts but on a philosophical position. For instance, physiological reductionists and psychological determinists take the position that all human actions are determined, i.e., not free. This leads to the view that no one should be held responsible for his actions: that they are "caused" by physiological processes, psychological forces, or social arrangements.[9] Others, for instance the existentialists, take the position that all human actions are free. In their vocabulary, the word "determined" is similar to "unknowingly obedient." This concept might lead to the position that everyone ought to be held responsible for all his actions.

Neither of these positions has been adopted in criminal law. For the deterministic position would lead in practice to no one's being held responsible for criminal actions; and the existential position would lead in practice, to everyone's being held responsible for criminal actions. In criminal law, the position is taken that men sometimes act freely (with intent) and at other times they do not. In the former case responsibility will be ascribed and in the latter case it will not. This position is not based on scientific fact. It is an axiom, the merits of which are argued on the grounds of its social consequences and social utility. It is based on the argument that justice and the common good are not served either by punishing all lawbreakers or by punishing none, but only by punishing those who are blameworthy and by attributing blame only where there is intent (or negligence).

The significant issue in criminal law, therefore, is not a scientific or technical question of who *is* and who *is not* responsible; it is a legal and moral question of who *should* and who *should not* be punished. As a question of law, the determination of responsibility is governed by legal rules (or conventions) that specify the circumstances in which intent should be considered to be present or absent and, therefore, under which responsibility shall be ascribed or negated.

Responsibility as a Legal and Social Judgment

In its legal sense, the word "responsibility" does not describe or refer to anything. It is a legal judgment made by one party of another and is similar to an act of giving, bestowing, and entitling.[10] The sociolegal matrix in which the word "responsibility" is used gives that term the significance of "accountability." This word has a situational or game-playing significance, rather than a mentalistic or psychological significance, which means something like: the judged eligibility of a defendant legally to be punished, which, in turn, is based on a judgment about the manner in which he behaves.

The criteria for the ascription of criminal responsibility are established by the specific legal tests. For instance, in the M'Naghton test the rules state that a man will be presumed to have behaved responsibly unless it is

> . . . clearly proved that at the time of committing the act, the party accused was labouring under such a defect of reason from disease of the mind, as to not know the

nature and quality of the act he was doing; or if he did
know it that he did not know that what he was doing
was wrong.[11]

The M'Naghton test is not a statement about human
nature. It establishes a set of rules for the use of the adverbs
"responsibly" and "nonresponsibly." These rules express
the ancient principle of English Common Law that a man
must intend to commit a criminal act for him to be punishable. They prescribe that a man will be judged to have acted
nonresponsibly if he acted without intent, and he will be
judged to have acted without intent if he did not know what
he was doing at the time or that it was wrong.

The M'Naghton Rule places the task of determining responsibility on an interpretation of the linguistic rules governing the use of the verb "to know." The use of the mentalistic
verb "to know" in tests of criminal responsibility disposes us
to reconceptualize the problem as psychological rather than
legal—as a problem of discovering the presence or absence of
a mental quality, rather than as a problem of applying the
rules governing the use of the words "responsibility," "intent,"
and "to know." This paves the way for the entrance of the
psychiatric expert into the courtroom to assist in the determination of responsibility. What can the psychiatrist contribute to this determination as it is governed by the
M'Naghton Rule?

What Does the Psychiatrist Contribute to the Determination of Criminal Responsibility According to M'Naghton's Rule?

The psychiatrist's capacity as an expert witness is based
on the assumption that he has *special* knowledge or *special*
skills (or both) that enable him to collect and appraise the
evidence for his conclusions that the defendant did or did not
know the nature and quality of his act or that it was wrong.
Accordingly, he is considered to be in a class with such other

scientific experts as the toxicologist. It is instructive to compare the operations of these two professions. The toxicologist possesses special knowledge in the fields of chemistry, pharmacology, and pathology, and he is skilled in the special techniques for determining the qualitative and quantitative chemical composition of body tissues. The term "special" indicates that this skill and knowledge are possessed only by persons who have had a particular training and education. Thus, the toxicologist can answer the question of whether a person had taken a lethal dose of arsenic. By utilizing his knowledge of analytic chemistry to determine the presence and quantity of arsenic in the blood and by using his knowledge of pharmacology and pathology, he may assess the likelihood that the determined amount of arsenic was fatal.

Much like the toxicologist, the psychiatrist is considered to be a scientific expert. Thus, it is presumed that the psychiatrist has special skills and knowledge that enable him to examine the mind to determine the presence or absence of certain knowledge, as the toxicologist examines the blood to determine the presence or absence of certain drugs. However, there are important differences between the psychiatrist and the toxicologist.

The psychiatrist, to answer the question "Does Mr. Jones know x?" uses the technique of interviewing. Interviewing uses linguistic and nonlinguistic communications, which (unlike chemical tests) each of us uses daily without special training. Interviewing may be defined as the art of conversation with the special purpose of obtaining information. Although interviewing may differ in certain respects from ordinary social conversation, it is neither a medical technique nor an exclusively psychiatric technique. It is frequently and successfully used in many other occupations—law, police investigation, personnel management, education, military intelligence, and so on. Labelling the psychiatric interview a "mental examination" gives it the sound of a scientific procedure, like the examination of blood. However, the toxicological examination of blood requires special bioanalytic tools and skills. There is a great difference between an interview of or conversation with a person and a scientific examination of a physical object.

The psychiatrist, in addition to using an ordinary technique, makes an ordinary determination. The determination that "Mr. Jones knows x" is a common determination that most of us make daily. Every day parents determine whether their children know where their belongings are, teachers determine whether their students know their lessons, and policemen determine whether witnesses know what happened at the scene of a crime. It is an ordinary determination because it is based on the use of ordinary language. Most persons know the situations in which it is appropriate to say "Mr. Jones knows x" and the situations in which it is appropriate to say "Mr. Jones does not know x." On the other hand, a judgment about the blood level of arsenic is based on an understanding of the special subjects of chemistry and pathology.

The use of the verb *to know* is based on knowledge about (or skill in) the use of language. This requires not only a knowledge of syntax, of rules of grammar, but also of the situations (or contexts) in which and the purposes for which words are used. Moreover, the use of the verb *to know* is not based on a knowledge of another man's mind. It is a commentary about his behavior on the basis of which we construct statements about his mental qualities.[12] Thus, we consider that a man knows geography if he can *tell* us the characteristics of various regions. We judge that a man knows the nature and quality of his actions and whether they were wrong if he can *tell* us the details of his actions, the events leading up to them, the surroundings in which they occurred, the reactions of others, the alternatives available to him, the purposes for which they were done, and their conformity to moral standards and laws. We use the words "he knows" appropriately when we use them to refer to a behavioral performance that *conventionally counts as knowing.* Conversely, we use the words "he does not know" appropriately when we use them to refer to a behavioral performance that *conventionally counts as not knowing*.

It is obvious that the use of these words is easy at the extremes. If a defendant can satisfactorily answer all our questions about the history, purposes, details, and circumstances of his actions then we are entitled to say, *by convention*, that he knows all he is required to know to be judged responsible. On the other hand, if the defendant cannot answer our questions, or if his answers are in obvious contradiction to independently known facts about his actions, we are entitled to say, *by convention*, that he does not know the nature and quality of his acts and, according to the M'Naghton Rule, is not responsible for his actions.

The use of these words is vague and ambiguous in the middle ground. If a student answers half of his examination questions correctly are we to say that he knows or does not know his subject? If a defendant can tell us about most of his actions are we to say that he knows or does not know the nature of his acts? The M'Naghton Rule does not specify how much about his actions a person must know to be held responsible; the Rule relies on the general rules of language for this determination.

The general rules of language do not specify how much a man must know for the words "he knows" to be properly applied. Knowledge about human nature is not relevant to this determination because at stake is not the discovery of a mental state of "having knowledge of" analogous to the bodily state of having arsenic in the blood but knowing the conditions of social behavior in which the phrases "he knows" or "he does not know" would be appropriately used. Psychiatric theoies are of no instrumental use in this situation because they do not supply the missing rules for the use of the verb "to know" in ambiguous situations. Nor will more information about the defendant's life history be of help.[13]

The problem of ambiguous cases is that the rules of ordinary language are ambiguous. It is not possible to resolve this problem scientifically since a further convention for the use of ordinary language is required. Nor could we hope to resolve all conceivable borderline cases by rules fixed once and for all. Thus, in these tests of responsibility, the rules are flexible enough to permit either judgment in most cases. This is one reason that psychiatric expert witnesses so often give conflicting opinions in courtroom testimony.

Jurists seem to be mystified by the language of the mind and to be unwilling to interpret the ambiguous language of their own legal tests. The legal profession seems to be under the impression that what is required to interpret these tests is special knowledge of psychology rather than a willingness to use vague and ambiguous terms. Thus, they turn to the psychiatric "expert" witness to assist the court in the determination of responsibility. However, in these cases, the psychiatrist either *must* interpret the language of the test that governs the determination at which he is testifying, or *must* supply his own criteria of nonresponsibility, which, strictly speaking, are irrelevant, since the determination of responsibility is a legal and not a medical procedure governed by legal and not psychiatric rules. In the former case, the psychiatrist serves not as a scientific expert, but as a linguistic arbiter who gives his personal opinion about whether the defendant *knows* the nature, quality, and wrongfulness of his deed. In the latter case, he serves to subvert the authority of the court by replacing the legal test of criminal responsibility with his own psychiatric test. In either case, the court enjoys the advantage of using the psychiatrist's scientific credentials as the authority for a decision that otherwise would rest on the weaker foundations of the ambiguous nature of ordinary language.

THE PSYCHIATRIST AND THE DURHAM DECISION

Over the years, dissatisfaction has been expressed with the M'Naghton Rule. Some psychiatrists recognized that the interpretation of this Rule is not a task for which they are particularly suited, since the Rule does not include psychiatric concepts. However, having become involved in these court-room activities, psychiatrists set about to alter the test of criminal responsibility so that it conformed more closely with their professional identity.[14] Proposals for new tests were based on the argument that psychiatric theory no longer holds, as it did in M'Naghton's day, that the formation of intent is exclusively the function of the intellect. Theory now maintains that intent is a function of interrelated cognitive, emotional, and unconscious factors.

The most important successor to the M'Naghton Rule is the Durham Decision, which formulates modern theories of intent in terms of the concept of mental illness. According to this Decision: ". . . an accused is not criminally responsible if his unlawful act was the product of mental disease or mental defect."[15]

Defenders of this test, and others like it, claim that it represents a scientific modernization of the law. They claim that it establishes as the basis of criminal responsibility a question of fact—the mental illness of the defendant—and they claim that it permits the psychiatric expert to testify about matters of medical fact and opinion within his competence to assess.

It is a mistake, however, to think that the use of the concept of mental illness in tests of criminal responsibility makes these tests more scientific. Statements about an individual's "mental illness" are not statements of fact. They are cryptic judgments that an individual's behavior is deviant and undesirable. The use of the concept of mental illness only seems to make the determination of criminal responsibility more scientific because these moral judgments are cloaked in scientific-sounding jargon. The use of the psychiatric expert witness gives only the illusion of scientific authority because of his medical credentials. Actually, the psychiatric witness translates his observations, explanations, and evaluations of the defendant's conduct into the pseudotechnical language of mental illness and health. He functions not as a scientist, but as the covert supplier of mental health rules upon which the defendant's liability to legal punishment actually depends.

Even assuming that the presence of mental illness could be established as a fact, the ascription of criminal responsibility is still a *legal* action based on the social and moral question of who ought to be excused from legal punishment. Legal tests and trials usually call for an assessment of facts. The determination of criminal responsibility is no more a technical and scientific inquiry because it is based on a question of fact than is the determination of criminal guilt.

Thus, in tests of criminal responsibility (and other courtroom tests)[16] that use ordinary language, the psychiatrist functions not as a scientist, but as a linguistic arbiter, who gives his opinion about the applicability of the language of the test to the defendant. In tests of criminal responsibility that use psychiatric language, the psychiatrist functions to covertly supply psychiatric values and standards for the legal determination of responsibility.

A COMPARISON OF THE LEGAL JUDGMENTS OF CRIMINALITY AND NONRESPONSIBILITY

The use of the word "criminal" involves a legal assessment procedure—the trial. The use of the term "criminal responsibility" also involves a legal assessment procedure—the determination of criminal responsibility. A comparison of the manner in which the assessments "criminal" or "noncriminal" and "responsible" or "nonresponsible" are made is appropriate.

The rules that determine whether or not an action is criminal are set forth publicly in writing. An individual may inform himself of them in advance and choose to conform to or violate them. Furthermore, the judgment of whether a law has been violated is made at a public trial, in an adversary proceeding governed by rules of evidence. The defendant is entitled to the constitutional guarantees of legal representation, confrontation by his accusers, public charges, and the right not to testify against himself. If he is found guilty, the penalty for his crime is established in advance and his right to appeal is reserved.

The rules that govern the determination of criminal responsibility, on the other hand, are vague and ambiguous; in effect, they are determined by psychiatrists rather than by law. The average individual cannot readily inform himself of these rules since they are expressed in technical language and vary among psychiatrists; therefore, he cannot easily choose to conform to or violate them. The assessment of responsibility depends strongly on the "technical," "scientific" judgment of the individual psychiatrist. His conclusion may be presented to the jury, but the basis for his conclusion need not be presented according to the rules of legal evidence. Although the defendant is entitled to legal representation, he usually does not have the right not to testify against himself. In fact, the primary evidence for the judgment of nonresponsibility is self-incriminatory; it is obtained from the defendant himself. If he is judged to be nonresponsible, no specific penalties are established, but he is, in effect, given a sentence of from one day to life in an institution called a mental hospital. Finally, there is no appeal from the judgment that one is mentally ill. One can enjoy a remission or a cure, but one cannot have the diagnosis "reversed" by a court of higher appeal.

Criminal trials are thus governed by two sets of rules: the rule of law and the rule of psychiatrists. The label "criminal" is ascribed when an individual is judged to have violated criminal law. The label "nonresponsible" is ascribed when an individual is judged to have violated the rules of mental health.

THE MEANING OF CRIMINAL NONRESPONSIBILITY

When an accused person is found responsible by a court, he is judged as any other defendant would be. He is either acquitted and set free or he is convicted and punished.

However, since the plea of insanity is usually entered only in open-and-shut cases of serious crime where no other defense is plausible, if a man is judged to be responsible he is usually convicted and sentenced to jail or to death. Thus, the term "criminal responsibility" (or "criminally responsible") is redundant. It means the same thing as the term "criminal," and its social meaning is legal punishment.

The situation is more complex in the case of "criminal nonresponsibility." If a man is judged nonresponsible, the verdict given is: not guilty by reason of insanity, and (in most jurisdictions) he is committed to a mental hospital.[17] Thus, the social meaning of "nonresponsibility" is psychiatric commitment.

A person who is judged not guilty by reason of insanity is technically excused. We cannot call him a criminal in the sense of a legally acquired status ascribed as the result of having been judged guilty of violating a criminal statute, because he has been found not guilty. Yet, every test of criminal responsibility assumes that the accused has committed an unlawful act. The M'Naghton Rule states: ". . . at the time of committing the act . . . he did not know it was wrong." The Durham Rule states: ". . . his unlawful act." The Model Penal Code states: ". . . wrongfulness of his conduct." Each of these tests, in effect, excuses a man for a crime of which he has not been convicted. The word "criminal" in "criminal nonresponsibility" therefore has the second meaning of that word, which refers to a person who is presumed to be guilty although he has not actually been judged guilty in a court of law.

The verdict "not guilty by reason of insanity" is semantically muddled. It implies that a man did not commit a criminal act (because he is found "not guilty"), and it implies that he did commit it (by the presumption of the tests of responsibility); it implies that he is excused from punishment, and it results in the loss of his freedom. There have been attempts to eliminate this ambiguity by separating the criminal trial from the sanity hearing. This in effect, separates the verdict of "not guilty by reason of insanity" into two verdicts: "guilty" and (but) "insane." In this case, the term "criminal" in "criminally nonresponsible" is given to the first meaning of that word, which refers to a legally ascribed status. At least this is more in conformity with the ancient legal principle that a man shall be presumed innocent until he is proved guilty in a court of law.

This, however, does not solve the dilemma of criminal nonresponsibility. The significance of "criminal responsibility" is that the defendant is judged guilty and is punished by being deprived of his freedom in prison. The significance of "criminal nonresponsibility" in cases in which the verdict is "not guilty by reason of insanity" is that the defendant is presumed, rather than judged, to be guilty and is deprived of his freedom by being committed to a psychiatric hospital. The significance of "criminal nonresponsibility" in cases in which the verdict is "guilty but insane" is that the defendant is judged to be guilty and is deprived of his freedom by commitment to a psychiatric hospital. In each case, the defendant is deprived of his freedom. In cases of criminal responsibility this is done by sentencing to prison. In cases of criminal nonresponsibility this is done by commitment to a psychiatric hospital.

If the consequences of the verdicts "guilty," "guilty but insane," and "not guilty by reason of insanity" are equivalent with respect to the loss of freedom, why are these distinctions made? If a man is judged not guilty, for whatever reason, why should he not be set free? If a man is judged guilty and deprived of his freedom, why should this not be defined as punishment? What is the social function of the distinction between the loss of freedom by imprisonment and the loss of freedom by psychiatric commitment?

In effect, the function of this distinction is to divide criminal defendants into two categories: those who are deprived of their freedom by being sent to a mental hospital and those who are deprived of their freedom by being sent to prison. In the first case, the action is based on the style of the defendant's behavior; in the second case, the action is based on his specific deeds. In the first case, the action of the court is usually defined as for the benefit of the defendant and is called treatment. In the second case, the action of the court is usually defined as for the benefit of society and is called punishment. To understand the social functions of this division—and therefore to understand the social functions of psychiatry in the determination of criminal responsibility—it is necessary briefly to consider the functions of criminal law.

THE SOCIAL FUNCTIONS OF PSYCHIATRY
IN THE DETERMINATION OF CRIMINAL RESPONSIBILITY

Four functions of the criminal law are usually described: first, to provide punishment or retribution against the lawbreaker; second, to establish penalties that will serve to deter future infractions; third, to protect the community from lawbreakers by imprisoning or executing them; and fourth, to rehabilitate criminals.

Early in the history of criminal law, liability to punishment was made to depend not only on proof that an illegal act was committed but also on proof that it was done with intent. Thus, certain specified conditions would excuse a defendant from punishment—mistake, accident, provocation, duress, immaturity, and insanity.

Of these excusing conditions, four may be construed to be unique environmental circumstances of which there is no reason to expect a repetition: mistake, accident, provocation, and duress. Insanity and immaturity, on the other hand, are believed to indicate a persisting disposition to act without intent, of which repetitions could be reasonably expected.

In cases in which the first four excusing conditions pertain, no purpose would be served by any of the forms of legal punishment. It would make no sense to punish a man for a mistake or accident for which he could not be blamed, nor for acting justifiably under provocation or duress. Similarly, there is no reason to establish deterrents for unavoidable events such as mistakes and accidents, nor for justifiable actions done under provocation or duress. Finally, there is no need to protect the community from, or to rehabilitate persons who, without intent, commit illegal acts under special, excusing circumstances that are not expected to recur.

The situation is different for the excusing condition of insanity. Two of the purposes of legal punishment are mandated while two are not. Since an insane person is considered to act without intent, he cannot be blamed—since blame is ascribed only where there is intent. Consequently, he is excused from punishment, since punishment cannot be given without blame. Also, it would not be reasonable to punish him for the sake of deterrence, since deterrence does not function where there is no intent.

On the other hand, there is the expectation that such a man "without reason" might repeat his crime. Therefore, there is a desire to protect the community from him and to rehabilitate him so he may be set free without danger to society.

To protect the community from an "insane" person, and to rehabilitate him, it is necessary to deprive him of his freedom. In all other cases, however, the deprivation of freedom is defined as punishment. If the insane person is deprived of his freedom, as is the convicted criminal, then it makes no sense to simultaneously claim that he has been excused from punishment! There are three possible solutions for this dilemma.

First, insanity could be eliminated as an excusing condition. Persons convicted of a criminal act could be punished and those innocent could be set free. This would require eliminating lack of intent as an excusing condition although other excusing conditions could be retained.

Second, a person who is found not guilty by reason of

insanity could in fact be excused from punishment and set free, as are persons who are excused from punishment on other grounds such as accident or self-defense.

Neither of these solutions has been chosen. Opponents of the first solution are unwilling to eliminate insanity as an excusing condition. Some of these are defense lawyers unwilling to lose one of their major defense strategies—the plea of insanity. Others are advocates of "therapeutic law" who believe that it is more humane to substitute psychiatric treatment for legal punishment, especially in the case of persons who are "mentally ill." Opponents of the second solution are unwilling to return to the community persons whom they believe are dangerous and likely to commit crime.

Pinioned by the horns of this dilemma that has been magnified by centuries of legal tradition, the law has chosen a third solution—the use of psychiatry and its medical rhetoric. The place of confinement of the defendant who is found not guilty by reason of insanity is called mental hospital rather than a prison, and the deprivation of his freedom is defined as for the purpose of treatment rather than punishment. This rhetoric permits the defense of insanity to be retained as an excusing condition. It permits us to consider the insane person as excused from punishment, and it permits us to confine him in order to protect the community and to rehabilitate him.

That the medical rhetoric of psychiatry disguises and resolves a *legal* dilemma is ignored by most persons for three reasons. First, it is a compromise solution that avoids the painful alternatives either of eliminating the long legal tradition of using the lack of intent as a defense for crime or of exposing the community to an allegedly dangerous person who has been excused on the grounds of insanity.

Second, psychiatric participation in determinations of criminal responsibility gives the impression that this procedure is based on the evidence and authority of science, rather than on the rules and judgments of men. The modern mind seems to believe that when moral judgments are phrased in scientific language they become less arbitrary and more humane.

Third, confinement in a psychiatric hospital in the name of treatment is viewed as more humane than confinement in prison in the name of punishment, although the principle difference between the two types of confinement is in name only. This view is enlightened only by the glow of benevolence emanating from the the medical model, which bewitches our minds to believe that those who act in the name of medicine always function only to relieve suffering and to restore health.[18]

The determination of criminal responsibility is not based on scientific facts about human nature or "mental illness." It is based on the legal tradition of excusing from blame and punishment persons whose criminal acts are judged to be unusual, bizarre, enigmatic, or shocking. The basic questions with regard to legal insanity are legal and social rather than medical, psychiatric, or scientific.

Most discussions of legal insanity fail to deal with these questions or deal with them only indirectly. This is primarily due to the interference of psychiatric jargon and concepts that obscure the legal and moral issues involved. This obfuscation, whether it is intentional or not, is one of the principal effects of psychiatric participation in the determination of criminal responsibility. It must, therefore, be considered as a principal function of legal psychiatry. The most socially important function of psychiatry in criminal law is to protect the community from persons judged not guilty by reason of insanity. The utility of this function is based on the ambivalence of the law toward persons excused on grounds of insanity. It wishes simultaneously to excuse them from punishment and to confine them for the protection of the community.

We pay a price for the illusion that psychiatric participation in the determination of criminal responsibility is scientific and humane. The autonomy of the law is weakened in its own domain. The interposition of the psychiatric "expert" between the law and those who are judged by it makes it more difficult for jurists to interpret and administer their own laws. The meaning of legal tests is permeated with an unofficial mental health morality that is obscured by scientific language and is therefore immune from intelligent criticism and discussion. When legal justice is replaced by "psychiatric justice" the Rule of Law is in effect, replaced by a "Rule of Experts"; and a "Rule of Experts" is simply a technicalized version of the Rule of Man.[19]

CHAPTER EIGHT

Community Psychiatry

Out of intimations of dissolution and insecurity has emerged an interest in the properties and values of community that is one of the most striking social facts of the present age.

—ROBERT A. NISBET[1]

The most recent innovation in psychiatric practices is community psychiatry—the so-called "Third Psychiatric Revolution."[2] There is no solid consensus about the nature of community psychiatry.[3] Nevertheless, resemblances to and differences from traditional psychiatric practices may be stated.

Community psychiatry resembles traditional psychiatry since both are activities explained and justified with the medical model. Like traditional psychiatry, the aims of community psychiatry are formulated, in part, as the diagnosis and treatment of mental illness. Like traditional psychiatry, its basic functions, which are disguised by the medical model, are socialization and social control; psychotherapy and psychiatric confinement remain the basic instruments for accomplishing these functions.

Community psychiatry differs from traditional psychiatry in the expansion of its rhetoric, aims, and practices. The problem of mental illness is no longer conceptualized exclusively in biological and psychological terms, but in terms of social evils and the social processes that produce them. The aims of community psychiatry have been expanded to include preventing mental illness and promoting "positive mental health." These aims are to be accomplished by means of early diagnosis, treatment within the community, and programs for modifying and improving the social environment. Accordingly, the activities of community psychiatrists extend beyond the traditional concerns with private and hospital practice. Community psychiatrists have become fully modernized and socialized. They have become involved in community affairs; they function in "mental health teams," and they employ techniques of mass communication to influence and modify human behavior.

COMMUNITY PSYCHIATRY AS A MEDICAL ACTIVITY
A History of Community Psychiatry

Community psychiatry is a complex social movement. Historians of community psychiatry usually attribute its development to four factors: public recognition of the neglected problem of mental health in the years following World War II; the increasing role played by the federal government is assuming responsibility for the health and welfare of citizens; recent trends in medical care; and new developments in psychiatric science and theory.

The retarded development of community psychiatry is usually explained in terms of long-standing public attitudes of "superstition, negativism, niggardliness, and unimaginativeness" towards the study and treatment of mental illness.[4] Interest in community psychiatry, they claim, was spurred by the beginning of the Civil Rights Movement in 1954 and by the subsequent recognition of the "Other America" of poverty, which aroused the conscience of the nation. Government has played an increasing role in providing for the health, education, employment, recreation, security, and general welfare of the citizenry. In the area of health, legislation has recently been enacted—for instance, the Hill-Burton Act and Medicare—as part of a "national program to bring adequate health care to all citizens."[5]

As purported medical specialists, psychiatrists have lobbied for a share of this new public program of health care. They reported to Congress that by 1955 there were more than 500,000 patients in mental hospitals across the land, occupying every other hospital bed and increasing their number rapidly. The total cost of these patients to the American taxpayer in government expenditures and loss of income was estimated to be more than one billion dollars a year and increasing annually in 10 percent increments.[6] As the result of overcrowding, it was claimed, psychiatric hospitals were strained beyond their capacities and could provide only routine medical and custodial care, and most psychiatrists ignored state service in favor of more lucrative and prestigious private practice and medical school teaching. Furthermore, it was stated that advances in psychiatry, particularly the development of tranquilizers and of social psychiatry theory, promised new, effective methods for treating mental illness, provided that funds were made available for research and treatment facilities.

In 1955, Congress passed the Mental Health Study Act to establish a commission to study the human and economic problems of mental illness, to assess current methods for dealing with them and to recommend improvements and new programs. Under this Act, the National Institute for Mental Health named the Joint Commission on Mental Illness and Health which, in 1961, published its report under the title *Action for Mental Health*. In February of 1963, President Kennedy proposed a "national mental health program" involving new emphasis on comprehensive community care to bring psychiatry into the mainstream of American medicine.[7] The Community Mental Health Centers Act of 1963 provided millions of dollars to construct new facilities for this purpose. This officially launched the Third Psychiatric Revolution.

COMMUNITY PSYCHIATRY AIMS AND PROGRAMS

Community psychiatry programs have four distinguishable aims: to minimize the separation of the hospitalized mental patient from and to facilitate his reintegration into his family and community; to obviate the need for hospitalization and to reduce the incidence of rehospitalization; to reduce the incidence, duration, and disability of mental disease; and to promote positive mental health.[8]

These aims are to be accomplished by means of four related but distinguishable types of community psychiatry programs: the modification of psychiatric hospitals; the construction of Community Mental Health Centers; the coordination and integration of mental health facilities; and programs to prevent mental illness and promote positive mental health. Each of these programs and the manner in which they accomplish the purposes of the community mental health movement will be described.

Modification of Psychiatric Hospitals

To reduce the isolation of the mental hospital inmate from his family and community, there is a trend away from the construction of the large, rural custodial institution and toward the construction of smaller units located in urban and suburban communities.

The older psychiatric institutions, which were constructed in large cities and isolated rural areas, are undergoing change. This change was facilitated primarily by the introduction of tranquilizing drugs into psychiatric practice in 1955. These drugs function as internal, chemical restraints that have a calming influence on thought and conduct.[9] They therefore permitted the relaxation of hospital security measures and a modification of administrative and treatment policies in the direction of the open door and the therapeutic community.[10]

In some older mental hospitals the bars have been removed, the doors have been unlocked, the patients are permitted greater freedom of movement, visiting privileges have been expanded, and, in some cases, men and women are permitted to live and mingle on the same ward. Some hospitals are modifying interior decoration to simulate home or hotel settings. Relations between staff and inmates and among inmates are managed by means of "milieu" therapy, group therapy, and patient government programs. Social activities are encouraged by means of recreational and occupational therapy programs.

The purpose of these changes is to make the hospital setting and the hospital routine similar to conditions in the home and community. This will ease the transition for the patient both when he is hospitalized and when he is released. Also these changes increase the access of the family and community services to the confined patient.

Community Mental Health Centers

The Community Mental Health Services Act of 1963 involved the federal government in a massive program to finance the construction and staffing of community mental health centers.[11] These centers consist of small, centrally located buildings that provide a wide range of psychiatric programs including inpatient and outpatient facilities; day and night care services; emergency services; pre-care, after-care, follow up, and rehabilitation clinics; half-way houses and foster home placement services; consultation and educational services; and facilities for training, research, and evaluating programs.

The function of these centers is to locate facilities for comprehensive psychiatric care within the community. By increasing the availability of psychiatric services to community residents, it is hoped that mental illness can be detected and treated before hospitalization is necessary. If hospitalization is necessary, separation of the patient from his family and community will be minimized and, upon release, his reintegration into the community will be facilitated. Also, staff psychiatrists will be available for consultation, and for educational and training programs. In turn, the psychiatrist may employ community facilities and resources to assist in the detection, treatment, and rehabilitation of mental patients.

Coordination and Integration of Mental Health Facilities

Community psychiatrists claim that the separate and unplanned development of public and private agencies dealing with psychiatric patients leads to duplication, omission, and inefficiency of services. Comprehensive mental health planning thus implies the coordination and integration of mental health facilities with one another, with ancillary facilities such as social welfare agencies, and with nonpsychiatric institutions such as courts and schools.[12]

The degree of community organization desired is illustrated by the following statement of a prominent community psychiatrist:

> This system [of organization] must include not only the governmental psychiatric services, both mental hospitals and community clinics, but also the voluntary psychiatric services and the other community services which are not labelled psychiatric, but which play a large part in preventing and treating mental disorders—the general medical services including hospitals, nursing homes, nursing agencies, public health services, family doctors; the social welfare agencies, the recreational services; the religious services; the educational system; the courts and correctional agencies; and so on.[13]

In this system of organization, the psychiatrist is to play a leading role as an organizer, an administrator, an educator, a consultant, and a therapist.

Prevention of Mental Illness and Promotion of Positive Mental Health

The principal theoretical orientation of the community mental health movement is that social conditions are crucial determinants in the etiology, treatment, and prevention of mental illness. The reduction of mental illness and the promotion of positive mental health are therefore to be accomplished by the establishment of broad programs in the health, educational, social, economic, and political spheres.[14]

These programs are directed toward individuals, families, and the broader areas of society.[15] They are aimed at improving education and employment; eliminating poverty, malnutrition, and other deprivations; providing recreational facilities; improving and extending medical care; interrupting "pathogenic" trains of events; and by generally ameliorating the stresses and crises of life.[16] One psychiatrist believes that "juvenile delinquency, school problems, problems of urban areas, community conflicts, marriage and family counselling, and well-being programs all can be seen as reasonably in the province of the psychiatrist, who formerly limited his interest to psychopathology."[17] Other psychiatrists envision the "therapeutic" application of their knowledge to prevent nuclear war and to reduce international conflict.[18]

This account of community psychiatry is heavily laced with the rhetoric of medicine, which obscures the history and functions of this complex social movement. The medical model influences us to view the history of community psychiatry as an alteration of professional practices due to improvements in public attitudes toward the mentally ill; the modernization of psychiatric theory and technology; and the modern, humane, and liberal plan for comprehensive mental health care for all citizens. The medical model influences us to regard community psychiatry as a medical specialty that offers in the field of mental health what medicine offers in the field of public health—the modernization of methods for detecting, treating, and preventing illness; the promotion of health and well being; and the increased availability of health services for all citizens.

This view of community psychiatry is too narrow. Community psychiatry is a social movement with a long history. Its development is related to profound changes in the character of modern social and political life—changes in national character, national purpose, and public policy.

COMMUNITY PSYCHIATRY AS A SOCIAL ACTIVITY
Another History of Community Psychiatry

Identifying psychiatry with medicine has obscured the long, intimate relationship between psychiatry and the state. The relationship between psychiatry and the community is not new; psychiatry has always served the interests of the community and of the state. In effect, the state gave birth to psychiatry by financing the construction of public mental hospitals. Later, the state financed and administered community mental health programs. Community psychiatry must therefore be understood in terms of the changing functions and policies of the state instead of in terms of the changing functions of medicine as they are expressed by the medical model. The transition from hospital to community psychiatry parallels a transition in public policy from one of confining and oppressing the poor to one of providing welfare programs for them.

In early Colonial America there were no psychiatrists, no mental hospitals, no public welfare programs, and no public provisions for the "care" of the "mentally ill." From the point of view of public policy, the class of insane persons was not differentiated from the class of criminals and of paupers. The term "insanity" was simply an informal epithet applied primarily to members of these two classes, depending upon the nature of their conduct. Thus, as Albert Deutsch states: "When insanity was publicly recognized, it was usually for the purpose of punishing or repressing the individual; when it was not, indifference to his fate was the dominating note. There was no unform theory for dealing with the mentally ill."[19]

The hospital "treatment" of the mentally ill in America, as in Europe, developed in the context of the social control of the deviant and the poor. Public attitudes towards the poor were harsh and laws were designed to repress, ostracize, and punish paupers. Initially, paupers were confined in prisons or, occasionally, were "boarded out" in private homes at public expense.

As the colonial population increased, public funds were increasingly allotted for constructing institutions to house poor and deviant persons. At first, these institutions were undifferentiated. The "Poor-House, Work-House and House of Correction of New York City" was used to confine criminals, paupers, and persons who, in retrospect, have been classified as mentally ill.[20] Gradually, public policy differentiated from paupers by the separation of prisons and almshouses. The "insane" were divided between these two types of institution depending on whether they were considered to be violent or harmless.[21] As Deutsch states: "The 'violent' insane among public dependents were ordinarily treated as common criminals, while the 'harmless' were disposed of in a manner differing only in severity from that accorded to all other paupers."[22] Gradually, the mental hospital evolved from prisons and poorhouses.

As in Europe, the inmates of these institutions were locked in unclean dungeons, hot in summer and cold in winter; they were often chained, beaten, taunted and permitted to rot and die from hunger, disease, and neglect. Following the French Revolution, a European movement to reform these institutions, especially the mental asylum, spread to the United States. These reforms were associated with a new brand of "moral psychiatry"—an intense, active reform program designed to rehabilitate rather than simply to provide custodial care. Deutsch describes the principle objectives of moral psychiatry, as practiced at the York Retreat, as follows:

> . . . to provide a family environment for the patients, as manifested in the non-institutional aspect of the building and its surroundings; emphasis on employment and exercise as conducive to mental health . . . ; and the treatment of patients as guests rather than as inmates. Kindness and consideration formed the keystone of the whole theoretical structure. Chains were absolutely forbidden, along with those resorts to terrorization that were still advocated in varying degrees by eminent medical men.[23]

While the principles of moral psychiatry received wide recognition, the most far-reaching and durable reforms occurred in private asylums that were primarily for wealthy persons.[24] Moral psychiatry failed in the public mental hospital, which continued to serve as places of confinement of the poor. Dain[25] states that before 1825 only two mental hospitals were completely supported by the state, and these served primarily custodial purposes. From 1825 to 1865 the number of public mental hospitals increased to sixty-two.[26] Thus, the mental hospital evolved along two distinct lines, each with a separate character and purpose, according to the social and economic class of the inmates.

The failure of moral psychiatry in the public mental hospital was due to a number of factors. In the nineteenth century the number of poor and indigent persons increased as the result of population growth and immigration. From 1840 to 1890 the population of the United States increased approximately 350 percent from 17 million to 63 million. At the same time, the population of mental hospitals increased by 3000 percent from 2500 to 74,000![27] As a result, poorhouses and mental hospitals were strained beyond their capacities. As the inmate population increased, conditions in public mental hospitals deteriorated. Patients were crowded into corridors or kept in barren, dirty rooms without adequate food, heat, clothing, or human company.

Although the originators and administrators of the early state mental hospitals expressed humanitarian motives and good intentions, their methods of dealing with their inmates were defined by public (middle class) policies towards the poor. Public funds and public instructions provided primarily for the confinement and security of asylum inmates and only secondarily for their care and rehabilitation. Psychiatrists themselves were drawn from the middle classes, and they brought the conscious and unconscious prejudices of their social origins to their theory and practice. The lower class inmates of state hospitals were poorly understood, morally condemned, socially shunned, physically abused, and psychologically humiliated. The interest of the early psychiatrists in neurology and organic theories of mental illness was reinforced by these attitudes, and in turn, these biologically biased interests fostered the treatment of patients as objects rather than as persons.

Although reformers campaigned for more and better facilities, as soon as new asylums were constructed they became overcrowded and the quality of treatment did not improve. Where reforms were instituted, they consisted primarily of reducing corporal mistreatment and improving physical conditions, which did not alter the basic function of these institutions. They still functioned to confine and control the deviant poor. "Humane reforms" simply led to the development of psychosocial techniques of control, instead of the use of physical force.

Gradually, public policy toward the poor shifted away from institutional confinement and control toward charity programs of support and care of the "harmless" poor in the community. Poorhouses thus disappeared and were replaced by social welfare programs. The development of community psychiatry signals a further shift in this direction. It signals a shift of the social mechanism for the control of the noncriminally deviant poor away from institutional confinement towards community surveillance and control.

This point of view suggests a different interpretation of the recent history of the Third Psychiatric Revolution than is given by the advocates of the medical model. For one thing, past public attitudes toward the mentally ill were not inappropriate. They were entirely consistent with the then current public policy to condemn, stigmatize, and ostracize the deviant poor and to confine and control them in prisons, poorhouses, and mental hospitals. For another, the present overcrowding of mental hospitals is not due to a contagion of mental illness of "epidemic" proportions.[28] It is due to three sociological factors: to the absolute increase in the number of poor and deviant persons due to immigration and the increase of population; to the relative increase of deviance due to the increased stresses of modern life on the individual; and to the increased use of psychiatry and the mental hospital for controlling deviance.

Once the medical model was officially accepted, however, it was easy to argue that mental illness was an important and neglected area of public health. The fact that mental asylums were called "hospitals" and their inmates called "patients" supported the claim that every other hospital bed was occupied by a mental patient and that mental illness was the nation's number one health problem. Using the medical model, advances in public health medicine were held as the standards to which psychiatry could aspire. The eradication and control of yellow fever, typhoid fever, and other infectious diseases were cited as evidence that with increased funds for research and treatment, "medical science" could eradicate or reduce the scourge of mental disease. The preventive programs of public health medicine were used as models for community psychiatry programs that would employ social measures to prevent mental illness and promote the positive mental health of the public.[29]

The introduction of tranquilizers into psychiatric practice, particularly into hospital practice, helped to convince a sceptical Congress that new scientific advances in psychiatric treatment were in the offing—advances that could dramatically reduce the number of hospitalized mental patients and thus reduce the cost of mental health programs. The discovery of a chemical "treatment" for mental illness was held to be a triumphant proof of the applicability of the medical model. Mental illness was at last "proved" to be similar to other illnesses because a new chemical treatment had been discovered. It was now promised that what antibiotics had done for the treatment of infectious diseases, tranquilizers would do for mental illness—if only the money were made available for follow-through research and treatment facilities.

The grounds for this new optimism was soon statistically demonstrable. After a century's rise to a peak in 1955, the patient population of mental hospitals began to decline. In five years, this population declined by about 6 percent— 30,000 inmates. This was offered as tangible proof to doubting and economy minded Congressmen that the last obstacle to new achievements in national mental health was the lack of funds.

These funds were now more important than ever, it was argued, because communities were being flooded with discharged mental patients who, having been dislocated from home, job and community because of their illness were now susceptible to great social stress and a recurrence of their illness.[30] Psychiatrists began to express the need for psychiatric treatment facilities in the community to help these individuals readjust their lives and to prevent or forestall a repeated hospitalization.

If we view the mental hospital as an institution of social control of the noncriminally deviant lower classes, instead of as a hospital for the treatment of illness, these events may be interpreted differently. Tranquilizing drugs have a calming and subduing effect on whomever they are used. In mental hospitals, these drugs calmed and subdued violent and agitated inmates, thus relieving the tense atmosphere of these prison-like institutions. As a result, security could be somewhat relaxed, hospital staff could approach and converse with patients without so much fear, and ancillary professionals and volunteers were more eager to work with inmates. Psychological techniques of influence could thus be used to persuade inmates to behave more in accordance with accepted social conventions. As inmates became less threatening, more amenable to influence, and better behaved, they were given greater freedom; they were given leaves, paroles and discharges.

In effect, tranquilizers converted the violent poor into harmless poor who then could be released from confinement. Just as social welfare programs replaced the poorhouse by providing social services in the community, community psychiatry programs are replacing the mental hospital by providing psychiatric services in the community. It is only now becoming recognized by the poor that the public welfare apparatus, as well as giving them financial support, has served to monitor, regulate, control, and humiliate them. Just as the harmless poor have been monitored and regulated by social workers, discharged mental patients may be monitored and regulated by community psychiatrists. This has not yet been recognized primarily because these functions are better disguised by the medical model than by the charity model.

The transfer of increasing numbers of "mental patients" into the community has required that the social control apparatus of the mental hospital be extended and transferred into the community along with the discharged patient. Thus, one of the functions of the community mental health center may be interpreted as an extension of the social control functions of the mental hospital into the community to insure that the discharged mental patient conforms his behavior to social standards of deportment.

The medical model facilitated packaging and selling "comprehensive community mental health care" to a willing Congress and President. The conscience of the nation was pricked by reminders of the history of neglect of the mentally ill. Medicine was already on the march and now advances in psychopharmacology had discovered a new "miracle drug" for treating mental illness. A newly emerging social psychiatry was gathering knowledge about the influence of the social environment on mental illness that promised to "sanitize" our social environment as preventive medicine had sanitized our physical environment. It was time for the planned obsolescence of the large public mental hospital and the construction in its place of the new community based mental health center to coordinate an all out war on mental illness. All that was needed was the go-ahead signal from Congress.

On the surface, viewed from the vantage of the medical model, it seems that psychiatry and government have joined hands in programs for the mental health of all citizens. Community psychiatrists, however, have not abandoned the traditional psychiatric functions of protecting the community from certain kinds of deviance, of regulating and controlling conduct, and of providing moral guidance. These activities have merely been expanded, modernized, and more subtly disguised.

COMMUNITY PSYCHIATRY AND SOCIAL CONTROL

Community psychiatrists claim that they have reversed the centuries-old practice of removing the "mentally ill" from their community by confinement in psychiatric hospitals. Instead, they claim, the mental patient is provided with an expanded range of mental health services within his community.[31]

Community mental health programs have not reduced the practice of removing the "mentally ill" from their homes and families, they have accelerated it.[32] The "liberalization" of psychiatric commitment procedures, which has occurred parallel with the development of community psychiatry, makes it easier to confine persons in mental hospitals by avoiding court hearings in favor of direct certification by physicians. Although confinement may be closer to home and for a shorter period of time, the number of persons who are confined and controlled by psychiatrists has increased.

While the number of patients confined in mental hospitals at any one time has declined since 1955, the number of persons admitted to mental hospitals yearly has grown. In 1964, the Department of Health, Education, and Welfare reported that since 1956, the mental hospital population declined 1.7 percent, but the number of admissions climbed 6.8 percent and the number of discharges doubled.[33] More recent studies confirm this trend.[34]

In spite of the modification of psychiatric hospitals in the direction of the "open door" and the therapeutic community, the social functions of these institutions remains the same. If individuals are admitted to mental hospitals against their will and prevented from leaving when they wish, these hospitals function like prisons, as instruments of social control. Tranquilizers and other innovations, such as milieu therapy and group therapy, simply increase the efficiency and speed with which deviant behavior may be corrected. However, this increased efficiency does not alter the basic nature and function of the process.

The rhetoric and props of the community mental health center make contemporary psychiatric coercion more difficult to recognize. However, the "voluntary" patient in an "open" mental hospital is as subject to coercion as the involuntary patient in a closed therapy hospital. The increased use of the voluntary admission route does not mean that more mental hospital patients are voluntarily confined. The patient who signs a voluntary admission form may do so because he has explicitly or implicitly been threatened with the longer confinement and greater coercion of involuntary commitment. Like the involuntary patient, the "voluntary" patient in an open hospital may not leave without the consent of the hospital authorities; he may be deprived of hospital liberties and privileges; he may be drugged with tranquilizers; he may be administered electroshock therapy without his consent and he may be committed for a longer period of time upon proper application by hospital authorities.[35] The fear of these eventualities is a powerful instrument for modifying behavior.

The "voluntary" patient in an "open" hospital soon learns to be interested in and "respond" to therapy: to avoid anti-social, immoral, or destructive behavior, to avoid disturbing other patients or members of the hospital staff, and to avoid any actions or attitudes that might antagonize his psychiatrists, his family, or his community.

Community psychiatry has altered the deployment of psychiatric social power over poor and deviant persons. Previously, this control was exercised primarily by means of confinement in exile in large, rural, custodial mental hospitals. With the Third Psychiatric Revolution, the exercise of psychiatric social power has shifted into the community. This shift promises to extend psychiatric influence over an even larger segment of the population.

Community psychiatry follow-up clinics, half-way houses and outpatient services facilitate the surveillance and control of former mental hospital patients. Patients are often obliged to participate in these programs under the rubric of helping them to adapt to social life following hospital treatment. While these programs may indeed help the discharged patient to adapt to community life, they also serve to keep him under the watchful eye of psychiatrists and other mental health workers, so that if the patient repeats his deviant or disturbing behavior he may be controlled with tranquilizers or quickly rehospitalized.

Community mental health preventive programs enable psychiatrists to observe and bring under control persons who have not yet been defined as mentally ill. These programs are justified in terms of "early diagnosis" and "case finding." In sociological terms, this means that psychiatrists will attempt to exercise preventive social control over persons who are potentially deviant and who do not voluntarily seek psychiatric assistance.[36] Dr. Gerald Caplan, a noted community psychiatrist, has outlined this new psychiatric "service":

> [The community psychiatrist] differs from his traditional colleagues in having to provide services for a

large number of people with whom he has no personal contact, and of whose identity and location he has no initial knowledge. *He cannot wait for patients to come to him, because he carries equal responsibility for all those who do not come. A significant part of his job consists of finding out who the mentally disordered are and where they are located in his community,* and he must deploy his diagnostic and treatment resources in relation to the total group of sufferers rather than restrict them to the select few who ask or are referred for help.[37] (Italics added.)

Another community psychiatrist, Dr. Harold Visotsky, advocates that: ". . . a benignly aggressive approach should be made to reach out and seek these people rather than sit and wait for them to come through [psychiatric] programs."[38]

These surveillance programs are directed primarily at the lower classes with whom psychiatrists have traditionally been concerned. For instance, neighborhood service centers, which provide "psychosocial firstaid" are being established in low-income areas in connection with community action and in poverty programs.[39] These centers, like all other psychiatric programs, may indeed be helpful to the persons who use them. However, as long as psychiatrists use social power to influence and control the thoughts, feelings, and actions of their patients, these centers as well as other psychiatric facilities must be interpreted as instruments of social surveillance and social control.

Community psychiatrists do not limit their attention to the lower classes. It has been suggested that psychiatric surveillance and control be exercised also over key persons in positions of authority and leadership who "exert a noxious mental health influence." Gerald Caplan has hesitantly suggested that these persons might be handled ". . . by obtaining sanctions for the psychiatrist . . . to intervene in those cases where he identifies disturbed relationships in order to offer treatment or recommend dismissal."[40] As psychiatric services interlock with other community functions, increasing numbers of persons from every social class will come under psychiatric observation and influence—including growing numbers of former mental hospital patients, mental health clinic clients, welfare recipients, juvenile delinquents, criminals, employees of large corporations, members of the Armed Forces, and students, as well as the families of these persons. Under the guise of providing psychiatric diagnostic and treatment services, psychiatrists who are employed by public and private agencies may function as agents of social control, as personnel managers, and as promoters of the middle class ethic.

Community psychiatrists often claim that their interest in the poor is a response to a public mandate for comprehensive medical care.[41] While there may indeed be such a mandate, it is unlikely that the poor have included psychiatric care in it. They have been the recipients of coercive psychiatric treatment for centuries. Myers and Roberts[42] found that the only psychiatric treatment with which lower class persons are familiar is psychiatric commitment, and they fear this to such a degree that they avoid contact with psychiatrists. Reissman and Scribner point out that this attitude is well founded, since ". . . all recent treatment census confirm the fact that the overwhelming bulk of blue-collar and low-income individuals are institutionalized when they exhibit mental and emotional disturbances, and are commonly regulated to custodial care rather than active treatment programs within these institutions."[43] Having defined themselves as physicians, psychiatrists have interpreted the mandate for comprehensive medical care to include psychiatric services. However, they do not provide medical services. They provide a modernized version of the control of certain types of deviant behavior by powerful community elements.

That they themselves may function as agents of social control has not escaped the attention of some psychiatrists. In response to his suggestion that psychiatrists exercise surveillance over key persons in the community, Gerald Caplan observes: "Such a role would be distasteful to most psychia-

trists because it places them in the position of a police de-
tective or spy . . . if psychiatrists did accept such a role, their
image in the community would become similar to that of
the Gestapo . . ."[44] Is the psychiatrist less of a spy or Gestapo
agent, if he exercises surveillance over ordinary persons such
as "immoral" mothers, students, former mental patients,
mental health clinic clients, welfare recipients, blue-collar
workers and criminals? Would he not be functioning as
a "secret policeman" by doing as Leonard Duhl suggests:
relocating "agitating and sparking personalities" to permit
disturbed neighborhoods to "restore some sort of emotional
balance"?[45]

Traditional psychiatrists attempted to guide and influence
only their own individual patients. The community psychiatrist works within such organizations as government agencies,
schools, and business corporations. By consulting with the
leadership of these organizations, he is able to influence
policy in a direction he believes will reduce mental illness and
promote positive mental health. One method of group influence is called by Gerald Caplan "Program-Centered Administrative Consultation":

> In this consultation, the mental health specialist is
> asked for help in those problems of administration
> which may influence the mental health or personal ef-
> fectiveness of personnel or recipients of the program.
> . . . The mental health specialist may be able to help
> the administrators maintain or raise the productivity of
> their institution while improving the mental health
> potential of the workers.[46]

A related form of influence, called "Consultee-Centered Administrative Consultation" is designed ". . . to help consultees
master problems in the planning and maintenance of programs for the prevention and control of mental disorder and
in the interpersonal aspects of agency operation."[47]

The community psychiatrist is no more a physician than
was his predecessor. The distinctive kind of help offered by

the community psychiatrist must be understood in the same context as that of the traditional psychiatrist—in terms of personal guidance and consolation. Only the techniques are different. The psychiatrist who observes an individual without his direct consent serves the purposes of social control no less than does a spy, albeit disguised as a physician. The psychiatrist who attempts coercively to modify an individual's thought, feelings, or behavior, or who detains an individual against his will in a mental hospital serves the purposes of social control no less than do the policeman and the warden. Community psychiatry differs from tradition psychiatry only in that its social functions are no longer exercised only in the limited arena of the mental hospital and the consulting room, but have been extended into almost every quarter of community life.

Just as the psychiatric control of deviance has been modernized to conform with present trends toward community social action, the traditional psychiatric practice of personal guidance has also been modernized to conform with modern techniques of public relations, mass production, and mass communication. Gerald Caplan recommends that the directors of preventive psychiatry programs employ full-time or part-time public relations experts to advertise the aims of their programs, to present a good image of the community psychiatrist, and to ensure the appropriate flow of clients.[48] The community mental health message is also relayed to the public by advertisements in the mass media, and the NIMH has allotted special funds for training mental health journalists.

Community psychiatry must be understood not only in terms of a complex society's needs for institutionalized procedures to palliate personal and social troubles, but also in terms of changing patterns of social power and personnel management. That community psychiatry is sponsored and financed by the state, and that community psychiatrists are the paid employees of the state rather than of their individual patients, suggests that community psychiatry is grounded in the ideology of the group. The self-defined interests of the individual will be respected only when they do not conflict with those of the group.[49] When the psychiatrist believes that his patient's behavior is or might become antisocial or immoral, the psychiatrist will employ his social power to restrain, confine or otherwise coerce the individual to conform his conduct to social norms.[50]

Psychiatric power, as an instrument of the group, is particularly well suited for use against the individual. Since groups cannot be defined as mentally ill nor be committed, they are safe from psychiatric power. In operation as opposed to theory, psychiatric power can have only an antiindividualistic ideology and, unlike other political ideologies, constitutes no direct threat to the state. Thus, the term "community" in community psychiatry is misleading, for the attentions and energies of community psychiatrists are directed ultimately at the individual.

COMMUNITY PSYCHIATRY AND SOCIAL SCIENCE

Allegedly, one of the major influences on the development of community psychiatry is the recent emergence of sophisticated social science theory and methods, which relate social and cultural factors to individual behavior, particularly to behavior labelled "mentally ill." Zwerling defines social psychiatry as ". . . the psychiatric study of man in his total environment. In general usage, it has come to represent the the theoretic or conceptual framework for the concurrent study of social and individual determinants of mental illness and recovery from illness."[51]

It is true that a significant body of social science research has emerged in recent decades. It is also true that psychiatrists have followed and participated in this research. It does not follow, however, that recent developments in the social sciences have contributed to the emergence of community psychiatry. To claim that this is the case is to ignore the impact of social events on psychiatric practices and psychiatric thought.

Theories relating social environment and human behavior, including "mentally ill" behavior, are not new. George Rosen has summarized views on the relationship between social stress and mental disorder from the eighteenth century to the present.[52] He reminds us that during the Enlightenment it was common belief that human well-being depended upon harmonious relationships with the physical and social environment, and that for the social environment to promote good health, it must consist of good social institutions. This belief was held by a number of physicians and psychiatrists of the day including Philippe Pinel, Benjamin Rush, Hack Tuke, and Rudolph Virchow. Many psychiatric theorists of the era of moral psychiatry sound very much like the social psychiatrists of today who emphasize the importance of social environment for mental health and mental disorder.

Why did not a vigorous social and community psychiatry emerge in the eighteenth or nineteenth century? About this one can only speculate. Certainly, the increased volume and wide circulation of contemporary social science research is a partial explanation. However, as Rosen correctly suggests, this question must be treated as a problem in the sociology of knowledge. Psychiatric theory has undergone transformations that are parasitical on transformations in psychiatric practices, which, in turn, are suited to the social, economic, and political temper of the times.

This transformation of psychiatric thought is illustrated by the following paragraph from the Group For The Advancement of Psychiatry's report on the preclinical teaching of psychiatry.

> The discipline defined as "modern psychiatry" appears to us a development which can be reviewed in the perspective of three identifiable phases. In the first phase, the psychiatric patient was viewed as an object; the focus of interest was biologic with the accent on observation, description and classification. In the second phase, the patient was looked upon as an individual with his own intrinsic economy, his own psychody-

namics. In the third and present phase, the patient is beginning to be seen not only as an individual, but also as an integral unit of society, in part the product of his environment and in part an agent capable of adapting to and influencing his environment.[53]

The three phases of psychiatric thought are related to three distinct types of public and psychiatric policies toward persons defined as mentally ill. The first phase of psychiatric thought flourished during the eighteenth and nineteenth centuries under a public policy of state-sponsored repression of the poor. This was the era of the poorhouse and the insane asylum, constructed with the "charitable" donations of wealthy merchants and class-conscious legislatures. Into these institutions were herded the dangerous and violent members of the poor and minority classes who threatened to upset the tranquility, stability, and domination of the small, thriving middle and upper classes.

Psychiatry responded to this policy by developing theories and practices that facilitated performing and rationalizing the mandate task.[54] There was no desire to alleviate the social conditions that "caused" mental disorder, nor was there a desire to improve the lot of the poor. There was therefore, no call to look beyond the poor "mad" inmate to the social origins of his poverty, his imprisonment, his despondency, his ignorance, his frustration, or his rebelliousness. There was primarily a desire to confine and control those unfortunate individuals who threatened the existing social order and the status quo of social relations.

Consequently, in the first phase of psychiatric theory, it was quite sufficient to view the mental patient as an object to be described and classified as is an animal in a zoo. Psychiatric theorists described, classified, and cataloged the "mental diseases," they studied the brains of deceased asylum inmates in search of organic causes of their "madness," and they constructed grand explanations in terms of phantom entities and forces. From the point of view of public policy, this theoretical orientation served quite well to justify confining, coercing, and punishing the deviant poor in the name of their mental health. Patterns of financing psychiatric thinkers contributed to the success of this theoretical orientation. There were no public funds available to pay psychiatrists to develop social theories and community programs. Consequently, psychiatrists drifted into hospital service and private practice and developed theories that explained and justified their functions in these settings.

The second phase of psychiatric theory is associated with Freudian psychoanalysis. Freud's theories are unique in that they take into account the individual with ". . . his own intrinsic economy, his own psychodynamics." This is because, in contrast with most of his colleagues, Freud practiced privately, and he treated exclusively patients from the middle and upper classes. He perceived these patients according to prevalent social attitudes as persons worthy to be listened to and respected. The fact that Freud listened to his patients and exercised no social power over them contrasted with the practice of hospital psychiatrists of ignoring their patients and of confining, humiliating, and repressing them. This single social fact best accounts for the distinctive quality of the second phase of psychiatric thought.

As public policy toward the poor and the "mentally ill" changed in the direction of state-sponsored welfare programs, psychiatry responded with theory and practice. The new order of the day called for the release of the poor from their houses of confinement, their return to home and community, and their moral, social, and economic integration into the group as producing and consuming members of mass society.

The development of community psychiatry is thus part of the national trend toward programs for the poor, the oppressed, and the dislocated. The modification of psychiatric practices in this direction required the modification of psychiatric thought. The conceptual need was for a rationale for programmatic action against social evils. The time was now right to incorporate the Enlightenment philosophy that man was a social animal whose happiness depended on the proper social and physical environment. Consequently, the concept of illness—of the locus for corrective intervention—was expanded beyond the single deviant individual to social evils and undesirable social conditions, which are the new candidates for psychiatric intervention and correction. Similarly, conceptions about the etiologies of mental illness were expanded beyond narrow biological and psychological boundaries to include social, economic, and political factors. The new theories of social psychiatry could now rationalize the joining of psychiatric efforts to treat mental illness and promote mental health with contemporary political currents of social reform and the quest for social Utopia.

Joining social psychiatry with government programs in search of the Great Society has altered the character of psychiatric thought and research. Just as patterns of financing influenced psychiatric thought in the eighteenth and nineteenth centuries to develop along lines conducive to hospital and private practice, contemporary patterns of financing are influencing psychiatric thought to develop along lines that will explain and justify community psychiatry programs.

The influence of government spending, and therefore of government policy, is likely to affect particularly academic psychiatrists who function within medical school departments of psychiatry. These departments operate clinical facilities for purposes of training and research. Many of them have applied for public funds under the Community Mental Health Centers Act of 1963 to develop community mental health centers. This promises to affect the staffing policies of academic departments of psychiatry and therefore to affect the character of psychiatric research, writing, and teaching.

An indication of the influence of federal money on academic psychiatry may be inferred from these excerpts from a statement by one department chairman:

> We are in a better position to receive some of these
> . . . funds simply by qualifying as a Community Mental

Health Center. . . . A vacuum baited with dollars is not long a vacuum . . . In the final analysis, I see Social Psychiatry as embracing approaches other than individual approaches, i.e., family therapies, group therapies, milieu therapies, social rehabilitative methods applied to groups. Clearly to expand our programs in these areas means either bringing in new and different faculty, trained in these approaches . . . or an investment of energy by current faculty in exploring, utilizing, becoming familiar with and assessing these techniques . . .[55]

It may be inferred from this statement that medical school departments of psychiatry will seek federal money to transform their facilities into community mental health centers and will selectively hire faculty to staff the programs for which this money has been allotted. The psychiatrist who refuses to practice commitment, who refuses to treat patients without their consent, who does not wish to participate in federally financed programs, or who has scientific interests divergent or incompatible with community psychiatry will find himself in an unfavorable competitive position in the academic marketplace.

The influence of federal money on academic departments of psychiatry is likely to influence the character of psychiatric thought. Psychiatrists, no less than others, tend to develop products for which they will be financially and socially rewarded, rather than products that are unmarketable or for which they may even be penalized. With an increasing number of academic psychiatrists functioning within government-sponsored programs and paid with government money, an increasing proportion of the psychiatric literature will be devoted to theoretical discussions of government programs. By the sheer quantity of this literature, theory congenial to community psychiatry—and, by inference, congenial to the aims and policies of the state—will be dominant.[56]

The medical disguise of social psychiatry has served to obscure the fact that it serves as an ideology to further government sponsored social programs. This may be illustrated by considering the furor aroused by Project Camelot a few years ago. Project Camelot was a study designed by the Special Operations Research Office of the American University in Washington, D.C. and supported by the Department of the Army. The objective of Project Camelot was to attempt to develop a social systems model that could predict and influence social change in the developing nations of the world. Specifically, it was designed to identify the potential for revolution, to identify the steps necessary to prevent revolution, and to determine how knowledge in these two areas might be used.[57]

Project Camelot came to an abrupt end within one year as the result of a complex series of events, one of which was American military intervention in the Dominican Republic. The connection between the Project and the Department of Defense raised suspicions in this country and in Latin America, that the research was covertly serving the purpose of military intelligence, to suppress revolutions from the left, and to support governments on the right.

Aside from criticisms of the research design of Project Camelot, the main criticism was directed at social scientists' conducting research for the Department of Defense. Some were critical of scientists who would lend their skills to advance the Cold War policies of the Pentagon. Others emphasized the danger that the goals and value-orientations of government-sponsored research might be disguised and obscured in technical language. Marshall Sahlins, an anthropologist, made the following comment to a national convention of his professional colleagues:

> . . . what had been for some time a cultural common-law marriage between scientific functionalism and the natural interest of a leading world power in the status quo became under the aegis of Project Camelot an explicit and legitimate union. In any event, revolutionary movements are described in Camelot documents as "antisystem activities," indications of "severe disin-

tegration," varieties of "destabilizing processes," threats to "legitimate control of the means of coercion within the society," facilitated by "administrative errors." Movements for radical change are in Camelot's view a disease, and a society so infected is sick. Here was a program for diagnosing social illness, a study in "epidemiology," called just that by a senior researcher. Another consistently refers to revolutionary movements as "social pathology," though disclaiming in footnote that they are necessarily to be avoided. A third conceives the growth of demands for change as "contagion." "Did the government," he proposes to determine, "couple limited and managed reforms with repressive measures to prevent the contagion and spread of social unrest?" Of course, waiting on call is the doctor, the U.S. Army, fully prepared for its self-appointed "important mission in the positive and constructive aspects of nation-building." The indicated treatment is "insurgency prophylaxis."[58]

Sahlin's statement is interesting because it illustrates that social values may be disguised by both medical and sociological language. Sahlin's statement is also interesting from another point of view. If social science may be used as an ideology to further the policies of the Pentagon, may it not, with social psychiatry, also be used as an ideology to further the policies of the Department of Health, Education, and Welfare? Is the ideological use of the language of health and disease to maintain the international status quo less scientifically reputable than the ideological use of the language of health and disease to eliminate poverty, slums, ignorance, and unemployment, or to control deviant behavior?

In both cases, social scientists are employed to further the policies of the state. In both cases, the value orientations of the state are disguised in technical language. Why has there been criticism of social scientists who work for the Pentagon or the CIA, but no criticism of social scientists who work for HEW? The extent of association of social scientists with the Pentagon and the CIA does not compare with the extent of association of psychiatrists with the Department of Health, Education, and Welfare! Psychiatric research is largely supported with federal funds and is often designed to promote federally sponsored social programs; but this research is framed in medico-scientific language, rather than in the language of morals and politics. Yet, there have been no voices from the scientific or psychiatric community raised in protest of "Project Community Psychiatry."

One reason for this, no doubt, is that the language of medicine serves better as a disguise for social values than the language of sociology. The intellectual community is somewhat more alert to the possible ideological uses of social science theory than they are to the ideological uses of the medical model in psychiatry. Another possible reason is that the elimination of poverty, ignorance, social turbulence, and personal unhappiness is a more universally held goal than the elimination of social revolutions. More people are thus willing to criticize social scientists for lending themselves to the suppression of revolution than for lending themselves to Great Society Programs. The issue being raised, however, is not the worth of the activities championed but the championing of them with supposedly scientific theories, which conceal the values and purposes they serve.

Psychiatrists and social scientists are entitled to take positions on moral and political issues. Indeed, it is moot whether they can avoid such positions and still remain relevant to social life. The danger to science is not that scientists will be concerned with moral issues, nor even that they will advocate moral and political positions. The danger is that these moral and political positions will be disguised in technical language and paraded under the banner of objective science as confirmed knowledge, which all who wish to be considered wise and good must believe. No moral or political values, no matter how admirable they may be or how universally they are championed, have the claim to logical validity or empirical confirmation.

As a science, social psychiatry is not concerned with understanding the relationship between man and his environment, but with changing it. It must therefore be considered an applied rather than a theoretical science, the goals of which are identical with the goals of the welfare state—to identify social evils and formulate programs to eliminate them. In this sense, social psychiatry may be considered an instrument of the policies of the state.

A greater danger to social science is that scientists will be swept along as a group in a single, unified moral or political position under the spell of a great leader, a great social movement, a central organization, or a powerful and generous state. The greatest danger to science is that it will be swallowed whole by big government and big business, in the service of some "ideal" social goal, so that there are only scientist-servants of these collectivities, and ideologies to justify them.

As much as the fact may be lamented, life is complex. Every plan of action has moral and practical disadvantages as well as advantages. If scientists unanimously support some programs and oppose others, there is the danger that they will ignore the vices of the programs they support and ignore the virtues of the programs they oppose. There is danger, that the methods of science will be placed in the service of ideology.

This has already occurred, to an advanced degree, in the case of social psychiatry. Few psychiatric scientists are critical of the aims and programs of community psychiatry, shun government sponsored research or service programs, abstain from treating mental patients without their consent, object to coercive psychiatric practices, or advocate other directions for psychiatry than the community psychiatry bandwagon.[59] Academic psychiatry has virtually become a subdivision of the Department of Health, Education, and Welfare.

The solution to this problem is not for social and psychiatric scientists to forfeit their moral conscience in the service of a fictitious "moral neutrality." Nor is the solution to abandon the use of scientific technology to achieve moral and practical goals. *The solution is to strive for frankness about moral and political values and to avoid monolithic formulations of any kind.* The cause of science, no less than the cause of freedom, is served by competing points of view in search of competing ideals and the means to achieve them. What is required of social science and psychiatry is not a unified—much less a disguised—moral vision for the common good, but a varied, critical, and refined perception of moral and practical alternatives for the common wisdom.

COMMUNITY PSYCHIATRY AS A COLLECTIVIST SOCIAL MOVEMENT

In its broad social significance, community psychiatry is, as its name implicitly suggests, one segment of the modern quest for community as that term indicates a coherent, ordered, integrated social system. It is one of a number of modern movements that attempt to alleviate the evils of unregulated, mass civilization by means of comprehensive, central social planning. In its basic design, community psychiatry is a thrust toward communalism, a search for elements of the primitive in the modern experience. It is the therapy of alienation. As a modern social movement, community psychiatry can be understood only in the wider historical context of the decline of community, the rise of the alienated individual, and the modern quest for community by means of collective social reform.

The ultimate goal of modern medicine is to reduce and eliminate suffering, disability, and death due to physical disease and, ultimately, to eliminate disease itself. This goal is a part of every modern program of social reconstruction. By contrast, the goals of community psychiatry are not components of political programs for social reconstruction; *they are equivalent to them.* Although community psychiatry first developed to control and reintegrate discharged mental patients into the society from which they had been expelled, the entire range of public problems that affect the life and well-being of individuals. Community psychiatry programs for preventing mental illness and promoting mental health are identical to the domestic programs and goals of the New Frontier and the Great Society. The prevention of mental illness means the eradication of social evils. The promotion of positive mental health means the construction of the Great Society. Psychiatric technology is a means for accomplishing these goals, and social psychiatry theory provides the justifying ideology.

According to social psychiatry theory, certain social and physical factors in the environment contribute to mental illness and others promote positive mental health. One of the functions of the community psychiatrist is ". . . to modify political and social policies and legislative and regulatory actions in the health, education, welfare, correctional and religious fields . . ." to provide "biopsychosocial supplies" and to help people deal with crises.[60] The mental health specialist seeks these social changes through consultations with legislators and administrators and by working with persons and groups to influence changes in laws and regulations. This kind of "social action for mental health" also involves using the educational system and mass communications to modify the attitudes and behavior of the community.

Among the social changes recommended by psychiatrists to prevent mental illness and promote mental health are: eliminating the material deprivations associated with poverty by such means as effective and humane city planning, slum clearance, urban relocation, and adequate housing; programs to prevent physical illness and enhance physical health; eliminating unemployment and improving working conditions, including employment regulations that would permit pregnant women and mothers time off from work; improved welfare laws, especially those that preserve the integrity of the family and dissuade women on welfare from having illegitimate children; improving the moral atmosphere of the home, including inducing mothers to marry and provide their children with stable fathers; providing education and guidance in child-rearing methods; improving the life of the aged by providing adequate housing, public education to reduce rejection, encouraging the mixing of the generations, providing part-time and light work opportunities, improving retirement laws, improving recreational facilities, and providing access to professional resources; influencing the educational system, especially to reduce unemployment and improve the quality of teachers and curriculum; improving efficiency and working conditions in industry; screening the population for "carriers" of mental illness and hazardous social conditions; and helping members of a community to organize to deal with common problems.[61]

Described in nonmedical terms, community psychiatry is a quasi-political collectivist movement that, by means of social interventions supported by state-sanctioned social power, attempts to palliate personal troubles, to foster the orderly and productive functioning of individuals in their communities and organizations, to alleviate certain disturbances of domestic tranquility, to organize and integrate community action programs, to implement the dominant social ideology and to promote the development of social conditions be maximally compatible with human desires and requirements.

COMMUNITY PSYCHIATRY AND THE MEDICAL MODEL

Like traditional psychiatry, the aims and practices of community psychiatry are disguised in the mantle of modern medicine. Community psychiatry is advertised as the psychiatric counterpart of public health medicine—as attempting to alter individuals and institutions in order to prevent mental illness and promote positive mental health. Like public health medicine, community psychiatry is sponsored, financed, and directed by the state; it is practiced in a group setting, and it claims to provide comprehensive "care" to all citizens, especially to the poor.

Like traditional psychiatry, the medical model serves to disguise the social functions of community psychiatry practices. It disguises the conventional practices of mental hospitalization and psychotherapy, which are still employed by community psychiatrists. It also disguises community psychiatry innovations in social control, moral guidance, personal consolation, and personnel management. Finally, the medical model disguises as comprehensive planning for mental health, the broad social values and ideals that community psychiatrists attempt to implement.

One of the most important aspects of community psychiatry programs is that they are designed, financed, and administered primarily by government employees. Community psychiatrists are usually not self-employed. They are paid by and owe their allegiance to local, state, or federal agencies. In contrast to medicine, where most physicians practice privately, the majority of psychiatrists, 73 percent, spend some time working for the government. Only 54 percent of psychiatrists spend any time in private practice and only 40 percent of these spend more than 35 hours a week.[62] The increasingly close relationship of community psychiatry to the state gives added significance and importance to its social functions. Previously, psychiatric practices were aimed at the poor—to control and supervise them—and at voluntary patients —to educate, guide, and console them. In its closer partnership with the state, community psychiatry has aimed its programs at a larger portion of the population and has widely expanded its functions.

Community psychiatry must be considered as a full-fledged member of the modern quest for community undertaken with the instrument of state power. The modern state is, of course, the most powerful instrument ever in man's hands for accomplishing good. However, as history had taught us, the quest for community undertaken by the state is the greatest enemy of the open society. There are indications that it leads, in varying degrees, to collectivization rather than to community, to homogenization rather than to individuation, and to obedience rather than to freedom and responsibility. As the modern method par excellence for controlling thought and behavior, psychiatry may well become the chief instrument of the state to bend the individual to its needs.

This danger from community psychiatry is matched by its potential for obscuring social problems and their solutions. The problems with which psychiatry deals are not medical, nor even psychological. They are social, moral, political, and economic. The solutions psychiatry provides for these problems are also not medical, but of the same nature as the problems.

There is a need to understand and solve the problems with which psychiatrists deal—problems of controlling human conduct, of reconciling law and morals, of dealing with the breakdown of the nuclear family, of providing methods of personal guidance in a complex social world, of healing the wounds of alienation, of reconciling the conflict between individual freedom and community solidarity, and of providing alternative visions of the future of mankind.

However, to the extent to which psychiatry becomes an important instrument for dealing with these problems, to that extent will psychiatry be the cause of our blindness to them. We shall be offered theory in inappropriate metaphor, so that it binds our minds in conundrums formulated in a disguised version of some prevalent ideology. The wisdom of the ages, which is found in all men to varying degrees, will be passed over as obsolete speculation, and the modesty that results from the admission that the truth is ethereal will be supplanted by the arrogance that so often accompanies monolithic dogma.

We shall have solutions for our human dilemmas proposed to us in the language of medicine, in terms of techniques for combating mental illness and promoting mental health, so that we cannot disagree unless we are wicked or mad. This can serve only those in power, who will promote their causes under the banner of medical progress. We shall have been bewitched by "experts" about our nature and our destiny. And this bewitchment will be eagerly sought by its victims—justified and exalted "In the Name of Mental Health."

Notes

For complete facts of publication, see the Bibliography. Shortened forms of references are given here—usually the author's surname and date of publication. The use of the given name indicates more than one author with the same surname. When more than one reference is cited for the same note, the references are in the sequence (a, b, etc.) in which they appear in the Bibliograpry.

CHAPTER ONE

[1] Mannheim 1929, p. 268
[2] Duhl 1963b
[3] Turbayne 1962
[4] Mannheim, *op. cit.*
[5] *Ibid.*
[6] Bridgman 1927
[7] Thus, the sociology of knowledge is the social science counterpart of the principle of operationism in physics. It is interesting in this connection that Bridgman published his work on operationism in 1927 and Mannheim first published his thesis on the sociology of knowledge in Germany in 1929. An historical study of the growth of these two ideas might well show them to spring from the same social processes, namely a decline in certain dominant modes of thought with a subsequent consciousness of conflicting concepts or ideas. In this case, the principle of operationism in physics may be considered to be a subspecies of the sociology of knowledge, namely the subspecies pertaining to our knowledge of the physical universe.
[8] Mannheim, *op. cit.*, p. 55
[9] For an examination of the social function of psychiatry in the schools see Leifer, 1969.

CHAPTER TWO

[1] Schiller 1903, pp. 9-10
[2] The term "psychiatric patient" will be used to refer to persons who are considered to be mentally ill.

[3] Although certain individuals with diseases of brain tissue are classified as psychiatric patients, they will be considered here to be medically ill since like all medical patients and unlike all other psychiatric patients, an alteration of bodily structure or function is the basis of their problems.

[4] Pleune 1965

[5] Szasz 1957a

[6] Popper 1934

[7] The psychiatrist who is most responsible for clarifying the difference between medical and psychiatric situations and practices is Thomas S. Szasz (Szasz 1957a, 1961a, 1965b). It is primarily because the description of these differences is viewed as an assault on psychiatry that Dr. Szasz is considered to be the foremost critic of psychiatric practices. (Davidson 1964; Bigelow 1962; Glaser 1965; Guttmacher 1964; Thorne 1966)

[8] Szasz 1961a

[9] Reichenbach 1947; Woodger 1956

[10] Morris 1946; Reichenbach op. cit., Wittgenstein 1953

[11] Szasz 1961b

[12] Parsons 1951a, b

[13] Parsons 1951a

[14] Szasz 1956

[15] Szasz 1965a

[16] Hollingshead and Redlich 1958

[17] This is in contrast to the use of the word "mental" in philosophy or literature where the term may refer to one's own mental events as they are "observed" in consciousness.

[18] Ayer 1956

[19] Ryle 1949, p. 16

[20] Bleuler 1965; Kety 1965

[21] Sandt and Leifer 1964

[22] Szasz 1957a

[23] It is also likely that when drugs are used for political purposes— to control the thoughts and actions of individuals—physicians will administer them, and their use will be disguised as a medical practice.

[24] Physicians, including psychiatrists, administer or prescribe huge amounts of medication to their patients (often at the patient's own request) to relieve their psychological uneasiness, to calm them or pep them up. When these persons take drugs, they are classified with physically ill individuals who receive medicine to cure their diseases, rather than with the mounting number of persons who self-administer pep pills, "goof balls," marihuana, and LSD to find escape from or solutions to the problems in their lives. The *basic*

issues with regard to drug use and "abuse" are social and ethical rather than medical and pertain to the problems of the social control and regulation of behavior rather than to physical well-being. Nevertheless, psychiatrists and other physicians usually discuss and advise about drugs as if their use were a health problem. This is another illustration of how medical rhetoric is deceptively used in the regulation of social and moral affairs.

[25] Tillich 1961
[26] Zwerling 1965
[27] Mannheim 1929
[28] *Ibid.*, pp. 255-256
[29] *Ibid.*

CHAPTER THREE

[1] Sigerist 1960 p.26
[2] King 1954 p.195
[3] Miner 1956
[4] Whitehorn 1963
[5] King *op. cit.*
[6] Cameron 1953
[7] Parsons 1951a, b, 1958b
[8] Engel 1962 p.12
[9] Kluckhohn 1949; Weiss 1949
[10] Bridgman 1927; Anatole Rapoport 1953
[11] Dewey 1925
[12] Goffman 1961
[13] Presthus 1962
[14] Goffman *op. cit.*, p.341
[15] Offer and Sabshin 1966
[16] Castiglioni 1941
[17] Bidney 1963
[18] Szsaz 1961b

[19] There is a broad consensus in our culture about what constitutes an undesirable bodily state. Most people value a long life, free of pain and disability. As a result, there are rarely conflicts between patients and their physicians about the need for treatment, even when the patient is not free to reject treatment. Most persons see their medical physician as an ally who will help them to achieve their goal of bodily health.

However, the situation is different in psychiatry. There is only a limited cultural consensus about what constitutes desirable behavior.

When a psychiatrist judges a person to be ill, he is judging that person's behavior to be undesirable. As a result of this judgment, a person may be deprived of his freedom and confined to a mental hospital. Under these circumstances, it should be understandable for the patient to consider the psychiatrist, who is the instrument of his imprisonment, to be his enemy.

There are, of course, voluntary psychiatric patients who may select their own psychiatrist, reject him, determine the goals of therapy, and so on. From the socioethical point of view, these patients are in situations similar to the medical patient. This, however, does not mean that the two kinds of patients are purchasing the same merchandise or being provided with the same service. It is therefore confusing to label both kinds of patients as "ill" and to describe both kinds of service as "medical treatment." (Tarsis 1965)

[20] Ellison 1952

CHAPTER FOUR

[1] Goffman 1961 p.379

[2] Ibid. p.264

[3] Zilboorg and Henry 1941

[4] Collingwood 1946; Croce 1921

[5] Redfield 1953; 1956

[6] Tonnies 1887

[7] Maine 1861

[8] Durkeim 1893

[9] Diamond 1963

[10] For an introduction to these typologies see McKinney and Loomis.

[11] Nisbet 1962 p.23

[12] Beqiraj 1966

[13] Childe 1946

[14] White 1959

[15] Ericson 1950; Keniston 1960; Seeman 1959; Wheelis 1968

[16] Burtt 1924

[17] Nietzsche 1885; Vahanian 1957

[18] Nelson 1965

[19] Devereaux 1939

[20] Ibid.

[21] This is the significance of Erich Kahler's famous phrase: "The history of man could very well be written as a history of the alienation of man." Kahler, 1957, p.43

[22] Benedict 1938; Goodman 1962

[23] White 1959

[24] Leslie White suggests that this difference is due to the fact that primitives were ineffective in dealing with vicissitudes of nature, but quite able to manage their well ordered social affairs. We moderns, on the other hand, have increased our mastery over nature, but find that our major problems are in the area of social relationships. White 1959, p.218.

[25] In the Middle Ages, three methods for guiding and evaluating conduct were associated with the Catholic Church: (1) the idea of conscience—by means of which explicit directives and obligations of attitude, belief, and action were incorporated by the individual as a sort of a moral gyroscope; (2) casuistry—by means of which perplexing moral dilemmas were resolved; and (3) the Cura Animarum—the cure of souls—by means of which confused, errant, and over-zealous consciences were managed. Together, these three methods for guiding and directing human affairs were known as the Forum of the Conscience and the Tribunal of the Soul. (Meadows 1966; Nelson 1965)

The Forum and the Tribunal are the forerunners of one form of contemporary psychotherapeutic influence, namely, that which is based on the social authority and social power of the therapist to hear confessionals, to inculcate moral values, and to recommend specific moral decisions in order to reform and rehabilitate confused, errant, and over-zealous "patients."

[26] Lowie 1920 pp.342-343

[27] Levi-Strauss 1955 p.386

[28] Radin 1927

[29] Radin 1937 pp.142-144

[30] Frank 1961

[31] *Ibid.*

[32] Fox 1964

[33] Durkheim 1915

[34] Brody 1960

[35] Henry 1941 p.561

[36] *Ibid.* p.563

[37] Foucault 1961 p.47

[38] Rosen 1956

[39] Rosen 1963

[40] Foucault 1961

[41] *Ibid.*

[42] *Ibid.* p.40

[43] *Ibid.* p.47

[44] *Ibid.* p.43

[45] Rosen 1963

[46] Foucault reports that the King of France believed ". . . . there are certain crimes which must be absolutely thrust into oblivion." He also quotes Malesherbes as saying: "That which is called a base action is placed in the rank of those which public order does not permit us to tolerate . . . It seems that the honor of a family requires the disappearance from society of the individual who by vile and abject habits shames his relatives." (Foucault 1961, p.67.) The keen listener can hear the modern state hospital psychiatrist say the same thing, although in the euphemistic language of the medical model. See also Rosen 1963, pp.237-238.

[47] Foucault *op.cit.* p.59

[48] Szasz 1961a

[49] Zilboorg and Henry 1941

[50] Pinel 1806 p.53

[51] *Ibid.* p.60

[52] *Loc. cit.*

[53] *Ibid.* pp.67-68

[54] Hollingshead and Redlich 1958

[55] Szasz 1966a

[56] Davis 1938; Leifer 1964a, 1966; Szasz 1957b,c, 1963, 1965a

[57] Szasz 1958, 1960, 1965a

[58] Breggin 1964

[59] Szasz 1966b

[60] Jones 1953

[61] Freud 1893 p.51

[62] *Ibid.* p.54

[63] The concept of the "functional lesion," which Freud invoked to explain hysteria, can be traced back to his earlier neurological work published in his first book, *Aphasia* (1891). In this book, Freud criticized purely anatomical explanations of aphasia in favor of a functional approach. (Jones; see also Breuer and Freud)

[64] Deutsch 1959; Szasz 1961a

[65] Holt 1965; see Leifer 1966c

[66] Breuer and Freud 1895 p.114

[67] It is indeed noteworthy that in spite of the legions of Freudian apostles who produced volumes of exegesis and discussion of Freud's works that it was only after sixty years that one man, Thomas Szasz, fully elaborated the implications of the differences between physical and mental illness. This extraordinary period of repression can only be attributed to the social value of preserving the medical model in psychiatry and to the professional hazards involved for

anyone who attempted to redefine the phenomena of "mental illness" as nonmedical.

[68] Fromm 1959

[69] Freud 1925

[70] Levitt 1960

[71] Freud 1927 p.208

[72] Freud 1926

[73] Freud 1927 p.207

[74] *Ibid.* p.209

[75] At the same time, Freud wanted to feel assured that the therapy would not destroy the science. (Freud 1927 p.209.) However, he was so successful in training psychoanalytic "scientists", that he glutted the market, so to speak. Psychoanalysts, no longer able to find a market for analyzing people, turned instead to trying to help them: to devising brief psychotherapies, to using drugs, to giving advice, to managing their patient's lives and so on. As a result, Freud's fears were realized. Psychoanalysts, in *their* pursuit of income, have abandoned the science for the therapy.

[73] Freud 1927 p.210

[77] Popper 1934

[78] Diethelm 1953

[79] Wheellis 1958

[80] In his classical paper on the neurotic character, Franz Alexander states:

The tendency which psycho-analysis has been showing of late is that of laying emphasis upon the patient's personality as a whole. This newer orientation presents the fundamental condition for understanding or therapeutically influencing that group of people whose difficulties manifest themselves, not in the form of a circumscribed set of symptoms, but in the form of a typical behavior pattern which is clearly a deviation from the normal. (Alexander 1930 p.292.)

[81] Becker 1963

[82] It may be objected here that one may attempt both to understand a person and to control and influence him. This is not quite true. The two tasks of controlling and understanding a person are mutually limiting, as the discussion of psychotherapy in Chapter Five will attempt to show. In any case, it is difficult to understand why a psychiatrist would attempt both tasks, since to control and influence a person it is necessary only to have power over him and to know how to use that power. It is true that the more *subtle* one wishes the control over a person to be the more one must know about him. This may be the motive of those who wish both to understand and to control their patients. However, this understanding

will be limited by the attempts, no matter how subtle, to exert control over the patient.

[83] Louch 1966; Peters 1958
[84] Laing 1967
[85] Becker 1963
[86] Jahoda 1958

CHAPTER FIVE

[1] Morris 1938 p.118
[2] Mental Illness and Due Process 1962
[3] Section 71 of the revised Mental Hygiene Law of New York State reads: "If the patient's condition at the time he presents his notice to leave the hospital is such that he does not appreciate his mental condition, and he is considered by the department to be dangerous to himself or others, another form of admission should be obtained." The "other forms of admission" (which are "obtained") after the patient has already been admitted) would permit his continued detention.
[4] Mental Illness and Due Process 1962 p.19
[5] Szasz 1965a
[6] New York *Times* Magazine, May 16, 1967
[7] Major Provisions of the New Legislation Governing the Hospitalization of the Mentally Ill 1965
[8] Mental Illness and Due Process 1962
[9] Goffman 1961 p.xii
[10] Adapted from Goffman 1961
[11] Hollingshead and Redlich 1958
[12] Tarsis 1965
[13] Goffman 1961 p.6
[14] Tocqueville 1836
[15] Goffman 1961 p.370
[16] Szasz 1961b
[17] Hayek 1944 pp. 72-73
[18] Muller 1961 p.22
[19] Elsewhere, I have compared the practice of involuntary mental hospitalization to a sympton of a neurotic conflict. In this sense, it is an unknowingly formed hedge—a compromise between our desire to protect (or better, to project the image of protecting) individual freedom under law and our desire extra-legally to control certain types of conduct.
[20] Council of the American Psychiatric Association 1967 p.1458

[21] Leifer 1964a
[22] Eaton and Weil 1955
[23] Parsons 1951a
[24] Mariner 1967
[25] Ryle 1949 p.46

CHAPTER SIX

[1] Freud 1927 p.210
[2] Noyes and Kolb 1958
[3] Shoben 1953 p.125
[4] Eissler 1965; Szasz 1965b
[5] Alexander 1931; Freud 1926
[6] The term "psychotherapy" will be used generically to refer to a general kind of professionalized personal influence. The term "psychoanalysis" will be used specifically to refer to a particular species of professionalized personal influence, which is here denoted as "educative psychotherapy." No distinction is made between psychoanalysts and other psychotherapists because these terms have come to be used more to describe an officially certified status than to describe a particular form of therapy.
[7] Freud 1927 p.104
[8] Jones 1955
[9] Oberndorf 1953
[10] Brody 1965
[11] Szasz 1964
[12] "Cost of Training Analysis Declared Tax Deductable." Psychiatric News Vol. 2, No. 3, March 1967 p.1
[13] Szasz 1964 pp.639-640
[14] Bennett 1965; Brayfield 1965a, b; 1967; Committee on the Scientific and Professional Aims of Psychology: Preliminary Report, 1965; Smith and Hobbs 1966.
[15] McMillan 1965, 1966
[16] Brayfield 1966
[17] Levine 1967
[18] In the sections that follow, a distinction is made between ethnicization and socialization. Ethnicization is the process by means of which the young are *directed* and *controlled* in the development of skills necessary to be a functioning member of a *particular* social group. Socialization is a more general term that refers to the acquisition of all social skills necessary to become a functioning member of a social group. Socialization is the more inclusive term. It is not

culturally specific; and it includes learning skills that may be deviant, innovative and creative. Ethnicization, on the other hand, is associated with direction and control, and it is culturally specific. The two processes are, of course, inseparable in the development of any particular individual.

The term "socializing therapy" is inappropriate since it does not connote the use of social power to promote specific cultural and subcultural value orientations, as does the term "ethnicizing psychotherapy."

[19] Devereaux 1956 p.15

[20] Becker 1962a

[21] Szasz 1966b

[22] Kesey 1962

[23] Fromm 1944

[24] Halleck 1967

[25] Menniger 1961

[26] Devereaux 1956

[27] It is remarkable that while ethnicizing psychotherapy resembles brainwashing in many of its features, most works on brainwashing or coercive persuasion fail completely to mention psychotherapy. This is an index of the success of the medical model in repressing the social dimensions of psychotherapy. See, for instance, Biderman and Zimmer 1961; Group for the Advancement of Psychiatry 1966; Hunter 1956; Schein 1961.

[28] Alexander and French 1946

[29] Becker 1964

[30] While the terms "schooling" and "education" are often used interchangeably, I prefer to reserve the former term for generic use to describe three distinguishable functions of the modern school: ethnicization—the molding of culturally specific attitudes and behaviors; training—the teaching of occupational disciplines; and education—the communication of information with no attempt to influence behavior. (Leifer 1969)

[31] Leifer 1969

[32] Szasz 1957d

[33] Leifer 1966a

[34] Szasz 1965b

[35] It is often claimed that whether they wish to or not, therapists communicate and influence their patients to adopt their personal values. It is true that the therapist cannot avoid making his personal values known to the patient. If the patient wishes to adopt them, that is his business. The therapist's business is to scrupulously analyze the patient's tendency to do this. The difference between

ethnicizing and educative psychotherapy is not, therefore, that the ethnicizing therapist imposes his values on the patient, while the educative therapist does not. The difference is that the ethnicizing therapist uses social power to impose his values on the patient, and he usually does not analyze the fact he is doing this. The educative therapist, on the other hand, does not impose social power, and the analysis of the transference consists exactly in the analysis of the patient's tendency to identify with and adopt the values of the therapist.

[36] Neumann 1954

[37] Freud 1930; Marcuse 1955

[38] Our society is both puritanical and deregulated. This means that there is an official prohibition of sensual pleasure. However, there is unofficially both opportunity and encouragement to enjoy them. This leaves the individual in conflict. For either he suffers from denying himself the opportunity for sensualism of which he could easily take advantage, or he suffers guilt and remorse for having taken this advantage. The degree of personal suffering caused by these social conditions should not be understimated. These conditions are the social counterparts of the psychological conflict which psychoanalytic theory postulates to exist between the "id" and the "super-ego."

[39] When we consider the influence of social power on the individual, we must take into account the influence not only of powerful persons and collectivities, but also of authoritative sociosymbolic directive systems and abstract values, maxims, and principles. Symbolic directive systems are enforced with actual social power; and abstract principles often function as substitutes for the explicit directives of powerful persons and groups. (Dewey 1920) This is why situated actions are vocabularies of motive: social contexts direct conduct. (Mills 1940) This is also why individuals respond to the directives of social contexts as well as directives of powerful persons and groups; indeed, the two are inseparable.

[40] Freud recognized that this schematization of the Oedipus complex was incomplete. In the complete Oedipus complex, the child loves and hates both his father and his mother. Freud attributed this ambivalence to the bisexual nature of the child. However, it is doubtful that the child's ambivalence towards his parents can be explained as the result of instinctual drives. It is more probable that it is due to the dual role played by the parents: both parents function as satisfiers of the child's physical needs *and* as the frustrators of those needs when they attempt to train and socialize him. (Freud 1923 p.27)

[41] Fromm 1944; Parsons 1958a

[42] From the psychological point of view, this transition from "paradise" to society includes the transformation of the child's index of well-being from the axis of pain-pleasure, which are "reports" on the status of the body as it is reflected in bodily feelings, to the axis of self-esteem, which is a "report" on the status of the social self as it is reflected in the attitudes of important others. (Ernest Becker 1962a)

[43] Becker 1962b

[44] Langer 1942

CHAPTER SEVEN

[1] Wittgenstein 1953 p.82

[2] Szasz 1965a p.265

[3] Leifer 1964b, 1967a

[4] Sachar 1966

[5] Szasz 1961c

[6] Grammatically, the terms "responsibility" and "nonresponsibility" are nouns that refer to states of being—to the states of being responsible and not responsible. But what are *states* of being? They are not persons, places, or things, as are John Doe, Syracuse, or stones. Persons, places, and things, however, may be said to be in different states. Things, for instance, may be solid, liquid, or gaseous. However, one cannot see, hear, or otherwise sense a pure state of being, as one can see, hear, or otherwise sense a person place, or thing. Each solid, liquid, or gaseous state is a state of some thing— a solid rock, liquid water, or gaseous oxygen. A state is a *mode* of a substance. To phrase this linguistically, "state" is the name of a class of adjectives.

"Responsibility" denotes the state of being "responsible" as "solidity" denotes the state of being "solid." What does the adjective "responsible" modify? It does not describe the state of a person's (the defendant's) body. It does not denote a state of his mind, since a person's mind cannot be observed. The adjectives "responsible" and nonresponsible" describe (or modify) a person's behavior. They function as adverbs, as functional equivalents of the adverbs "responsibly" and "not responsibly." This shows that the determination of criminal responsibility does not require an investigation of the presence or absence of a state of mind. It requires the evaluation and judgment of behavior.

[7] Ayer 1956

[8] Wittgenstein 1953

[9] One of the consequences of this position, which is shared by many psychiatrists, social workers, and liberal reformers, is that crime is conceptualized as illness. Accordingly, these persons recommend that criminals receive treatment rather than punishment. Some suggestions about the motives and social functions of this switch in rhetoric appear further on in this chapter.

[10] Hart 1960

[11] M'Naghton's Case 1843

[12] Ayer 1956

[13] The judgment that a defendant knew the nature and quality of his acts, or that they were wrong, requires obtaining information from him. The psychiatrist, however, has no monopoly on the skill of interviewing. Nor can interviewing be considered by any criterion to be a medical skill. A lawyer or judge could equally well obtain the information necessary for making a judgment of criminal responsibility.

[14] GAP 1954

[15] Durham v United States 1954

[16] For a discussion of the competence of the psychiatrist to assist in legal determinations of incompetence see Leifer 1964a.

[17] Davidson 1966; Haines and Zeidler 1958; Weihofen 1954

[18] Nice 1958

[19] Szasz 1965a

CHAPTER EIGHT

[1] Nisbet 1962 p.23

[2] The First Psychiatric Revolution, symbolized by Pinel's striking the chains from the inmates of the Bicetre in 1793, consisted of liberal and humane reforms in the treatment of the hospitalized mentally ill. This revolution launched the era of hospital psychiatry. The Second Psychiatric Revolution consisted of the introduction of psychoanalysis into psychiatry by Sigmund Freud and his followers. This revolution launched the era of private practice. (Bellak 1964; Hobbs 1969)

[3] Goldston 1965

[4] Gorman 1956 p.10; Zilboorg and Henry 1941

[5] Thompkins 1967

[6] Joint Commission on Mental Illness and Mental Health 1961

[7] Kennedy 1964

[8] Caplan 1964

[9] Szasz 1957b

[10] Belknap 1956; Cumming and Cumming 1962; Jones 1952; Robert Rapoport 1960; Research Conference on Therapeutic Community 1960

[11] Felix 1963; Kennedy 1964; Ozarin and Brown 1964

[12] Joint Commission on Mental Illness and Mental Health 1960; Perlen and Kahn 1963

[13] Caplan 1964 p.139

[14] Eisenberg 1962; Freedman 1963; Rafferty 1963

[15] Bolman and Westman 1967

[16] Caplan 1964

[17] Visotsky 1965 p.692

[18] Group for the Advancement of Psychiatry 1966; Meachum 1964; Raskin 1964

[19] Deutsch 1937 p.41

[20] In his classic book *The Mentally Ill in America*, Albert Deutsch reveals the influence of the medical model on his thinking. He states: "The individual in need of assistance was apt to receive public attention only when his condition was looked upon as a social danger or a public nuisance—and he was then 'disposed of' rather than helped." (Deutsch, Albert 1937 p.40) However, whether such an individual is in need of assistance or should be "disposed of" depends on whether he is defined as mentally ill or as socially deviant. The citizens of this period obviously did not use the medical model as we do, to describe certain forms of deviant conduct. They regarded persons who were socially dangerous or nuisances as deviant and disposed of them accordingly. Deutsch retrospectively defines these dangerous and bothersome persons as mentally ill and then complains because they were "disposed of" as if they were deviant rather than assisted as if they were ill. This retrospective application of the medical model prevents Deutsch from writing a social rather than a medical history of the treatment of the mentally ill.

[21] This division is visible today in New York State where the "harmless insane" are kept in mental hospitals regulated by the Department of Mental Hygiene. The "violent (or criminal) insane," on the other hand, are kept in institutions regulated by the Department of Corrections.

[22] Deutsch *op.cit.* p.41

[23] *Ibid.* p.94

[24] Dain 1964 p.51

[25] *Ibid.* p.52

[26] *Ibid.* p.55

[27] Deutsch *op. cit.* p.232

28 Gorman 1956

29 The mental hygiene lobby in Washington played an important role in the development of community psychiatry programs. This lobby successfully promoted the medical model for viewing psychiatric activities and successfully lobbied Congress for legislation to finance new mental health programs. Having succeeded in their lobby, psychiatrists then claimed that they were responding to a mandate from the people for these programs. (Thompkins; see also Bolman)

30 Cumming and Cumming 1957

31 Malamud and Braceland 1966

32 Leifer 1966b

33 "Community Mental Health Advances" 1964

34 Number of Mental Hospital Patients Drops 1967

35 Breggin 1964

36 Dr. Gerald Caplan has described one technique of preventive intervention as "anticipatory guidance." With this technique "the preventive psychiatrist gains access to a population which he has reason to believe will shortly be exposed to hazardous circumstances that will provoke crisis in a significant proportion such as a group of patients awaiting elective surgery, a group of children awaiting admission to kindergarten or college, a group of pregnant women before labor, or a group of Peace Corps volunteers preparing to go overseas." (Caplan 1964 p.84) While such anticipatory guidance may indeed be helpful to these individuals, it also affords the psychiatrist an opportunity to exercise preventive social control over individuals who, he believes, might commit deviant and disturbing actions in the future.

37 Caplan 1965 pp.4-5

38 Vistosky 1964 p.435

39 Reissman and Hallowitz 1967

40 Caplan 1964 pp.78-79

41 Thompkins 1967

42 Myers and Roberts 1959

43 Reissman and Scribner 1965 p.798

44 Caplan 1964 pp.79-80

45 Duhl 1963a, b

46 Caplan 1964 p.217

47 *Ibid.* p.227

48 *Ibid.* pp.208-209

49 Szasz 1966

50 Halleck 1967

51 Zwerling also mentions the following areas of social study as significantly influencing the development of social psychiatry and

community psychiatry. (1) The study of the mental hospital as a total community; (2) demographic studies of the prevalance of mental illness; (3) transcultural studies, which reveal patterns of incidence and prevalence of mental illness not easily explainable from the standpoint of individual psychodynamics; (4) sociological studies of motivational influences in small groups; (5) studies of the family as a social unit; and finally, (6) the work of ego-psychologists that emphasize the influence of social learning on individual behavior. (Zwerling 1965)

The sociological study of "mental illness," if it is sharply defined, is actually the study of persons who have been labelled mentally ill by psychiatrists. In these studies, the social functions of psychiatry should be at least as important as the social characteristics of the individuals defined as mentally ill. It is noteworthy that Zwerling, like many of his social psychiatry colleagues, neglects to discuss the sociology of psychiatry as a relevant variable in sociological studies of mental illness. One is tempted to conclude that this systematic omission serves to mask the social value which is inherent in discussions of "mental illness" and "psychopathology."

[52] Rosen 1959

[53] Group for the Advancement of Psychiatry 1962 p.51

[54] This response was unconscious in the sense that psychiatrists were unaware of the influence of broad sociopolitical contexts on their thought and action. They did not understand their theories in terms of the sociology of knowledge nor their practices in terms of the sociology of psychiatry. This is understandable since the full development of these perspectives did not occur until the third decade of the twentieth century. Today, we are able to position psychiatric thought and practice in a full social perspective.

[55] Robinson 1966

[56] Leifer 1967b

[57] Horowitz 1967

[58] Sahlins 1967 pp.77-78

[59] Dunham 1965

[60] Caplan 1964 p.56

[61] Ibid. Chapter III

[62] Lockman 1966

Bibliography

Alexander, Franz (1930) "The Neurotic Character," *International Journal of Psychoanalysis*, 11:292-311 (July).

—— (1931) "Psychoanalysis and Medicine," *The Scope of Psychoanalysis 1921-1961: Selected Papers of Franz Alexander*. New York: Basic Books, 1961.

Alexander, Franz and French, Thomas M. (1946). *Psychoanalytic Therapy: Principles and Application*. New York: Ronald Press.

Ayer, Alfred Jules (1956) *The Problem of Knowledge*. London: Macmillan.

Becker, Ernest (1962a) *The Birth and Death of Meaning*. New York: The Free Press.

—— (1962b) "Socialization, Command of Performance and Mental Illness," *American Journal of Sociology*, 67:494-501 (March).

—— (1964) *The Revolution in Psychiatry*. New York: The Free Press.

Becker, Howard (1963) *Outsiders: Studies in the Sociology of Deviance*. New York: The Free Press.

Belknap, Ivan (1956) *Human Problems of a State Mental Hospital*. New York: McGraw-Hill.

Bellak, Leopold (1964) "Community Psychiatry: The Third Psychiatric Revolution," *Handbook of Community Psychiatry and Community Mental Health*, Leopold Bellak (ed.) New York: Grune and Stratton.

Benedict, Ruth (1938) "Continuities and Discontinuities in Cultural Conditioning," *Psychiatry*, 1:161-169 (May).

Bennet, Chester C. (1965) "Community Psychology: Impressions of the Boston Conference on the Education of Psychologists for Community Mental Health," *American Psychologist*, 20:832-835.

Bequiraj, Mehmet (1966) *Peasantry In Revolution*. Cornell Research Papers in International Studies—V. Ithaca, New York: Center for International Studies Cornell University.

Biderman, Albert D. and Zimmer, Herbert (eds.) (1961) *The Manipulation of Human Behavior*. New York: John Wiley and Sons.

Bidney, David (1963) "So-called Primitive Medicine and Religion," *Man's Image in Medicine and Anthropology*. Iago Goldston, ed. Monograph IV, Institute of Social and Historical Medicine. New York: International Universities Press.

Bigelow, Newton (1962) "Editorial Comment: Sass for the Gander," *Psychiatric Quarterly*, 36:754-767.

Bleuler, Manfred (1965) "Conceptions of Schizophrenia Within the Last Fifty Years and Today," *International Journal of Psychiatry*, 1:501-513 (October).

Bolman, William M. (1967) "Theoretical and Empirical Bases of Community Mental Health," *American Journal of Psychiatry* (Supplement), 124:8-13 (October).

Bolman, William M. and Westman, Jack C. (1967) "Prevention of Mental Disorder: An Overview of Current Programs," *American Journal of Psychiatry*, 123:1058-1068 (March).

Brayfield, Arthur (1965a) "Human Effectiveness," *American Psychologist*, 20:645-651.

—— (1965b) "Community Mental Health Centers 'Staffing' Legislation," *American Psychologist*, 20:429-430.

—— (1966) "Report of the Executive Officer: 1966," *American Psychologist*, 21:1121 (December).

—— (1967) "Psychology and Medicare," *American Psychologist*, 22:444-447 (June).

Breggin, Peter (1964) "Coercion of Voluntary Patients in an Open Hospital," *Archives of General Psychiatry* 10:173-181 (February).

Breuer, Joseph and Freud, Sigmund (1895) *Studies in Hysteria* Boston: Beacon Press, 1937.

Bridgman, Percy (1927) *The Logic of Modern Physics*. New York: The Macmillan Company, 1960.

Brody, Eugene B. (1960) "The Public Mental Hospital as a Symptom of Social Conflict," *Maryland State Medical Journal*, 9:330-334.

Brody, Matthew (1965) "State Medical Society Opposes Unsupervised Lay Psycho-Therapy," *The Bulletin of the New York State District Branches of the American Psychiatric Association*. 8:3 (September).

Burtt, E. A., (1924). *The Metaphysical Foundations of Modern Physical Science*, rev. ed. International Library of Psychology, Philosophy and Scientific Method. London: Routledge and Kegan Paul, 1932.

Cameron, Ewen D. (1953) "A Theory of Diagnosis," *Current Problems in Psychiatric Diagnosis*. Paul Hoch and Joseph Zubin, eds. New York: Grune and Stratton.

Caplan, Gerald (1964) *Principles of Preventive Psychiatry*. New York: Basic Books.

————— (1965) "Community Psychiatry—Introduction and Overview," In *Concepts of Community Psychiatry: A Framework for Training*. United States Department of Health, Education and Welfare, Public Health Service Publication No. 1319.

Castiglioni, Arturo (1941) *A History of Medicine*. New York: Alfred A. Knopf.

Childe, V. Gordon (1942) *What Happened in History*. Baltimore: Penguin Books.

Clausen, John A. (1956) *Sociology and the Field of Mental Health*. New York: Russell Sage Foundation.

Collingwood, R. G. (1946) *The Idea of History*. New York: Clarendon Press.

"Committee on the Scientific and Professional Aims of Psychology: Preliminary Report," (1965) *American Psychologist* 20:95-100.

"Community Mental Health Advances (1964) United States Department of Health, Education and Welfare, Public Health Service Pamphlet No. 1141.

"Cost of Training Analysis Declared Tax Deductable," *Psychiatric News*. Vol. 2, No. 3, March 1967.

Council of the American Psychiatric Association (1967) "Position Statement on the Question of Adequacy of Treatment" *American Journal of Psychiatry* 123:1458-1460 (May).

Croce, Benedetto (1921) *History: Its Theory and Practice* Douglas Ainslee, Transl., New York: Harcourt, Brace and Company, Inc.

Cumming, John and Cumming, Elaine (1957) *Closed Ranks: Experiment in Mental Health Education*. Cambridge: Harvard University Press.

————— (1962) *Ego and Milieu*. New York: Atherten Press.

Daine, Norman (1964) *Concepts of Insanity in The United States, 1789-1865*. New Brunswick, New Jersey: Rutgers University Press.

Davidson, Henry A. (1964) "The New War on Psychiatry," *American Journal of Psychiatry* 121:528-534 (December).

————— (1966) "Psychiatric Examination and Civil Rights," Slovenko, Ralph ed. *Crime Law and Corrections*. Springfield, Illinois: Charles C. Thomas.

Davis, Kingsley (1938) "Mental Hygiene and the Class Structure," *Psychiatry*, 1:55-65 (February).

Deutsch, Albert (1937) *The Mentally Ill in America: A History of Their Care and Treatment from Colonial Times*, 2d ed., rev. New York: Columbia University Press.

Deutsch, Felix (1959) *The Mysterious Leap from the Mind to the Body*. New York: International Universities Press.

Devereaux, George (1939) "A Sociological Theory of Schizophrenia," *Psychoanalytic Review*, 26:315-342 (June).

———— (1956) *Therapeutic Education.* New York: Harper and Brothers.

Dewey, John (1920) *Reconstruction in Philosophy.* Boston: Beacon Press, 1948.

———— (1925) *Experience and Nature.* Chicago: Open Court Publishing Company.

Diamond, Stanley (1963) "The Search for the Primitive," *Man's Image in Medicine and Anthropology.* Iago Goldston, ed. New York: International Universities Press.

Diethelm, Oskar (1953) "The Fallacy of the Concept: Psychosis," *Current Problems in Psychiatric Diagnosis.* Paul Hoch and Joseph Zubin eds. New York: Grune and Stratton.

Driver, Edwin D. (1965) *The Sociology and Anthropology of Mental Illness: A Reference Guide.* Amherst, Mass.: The University of Massachusetts Press.

Duhl, Leonard J. (1963a) "The Changing Face of Mental Health," *The Urban Condition.* Leonard Duhl, ed. New York: Basic Books.

———— (1963b) "The Psychiatric Evolution," *Concepts of Community Psychiatry: A Framework for Training.* Stephen E. Goldston, ed. Public Health Service Publication No. 1319. Bethesda, Maryland: National Institute of Mental Health, 1965.

Dunham, H. Warren (1965) "Community Psychiatry: The Newest Therapeutic Bandwagon," *Archives of General Psychiatry,* 12:303-313 (March).

Durham v. United States (1954) U. S. App. D. C. 214 F. 2d 862.

Durkheim, Emile (1893) *The Division of Labor in Society.* George Simpson, Transl. 1964. New York: The Free Press: A division of the Macmillan Co.

———— (1915) *The Elementary Forms of the Religious Life.* Joseph W. Swarz, transl. New York: Macmillan.

Eaton, Joseph W. and Weil, Robert J. (1955) *Culture and Mental Disorders.* Glencoe, Illinois: The Free Press of Glencoe.

Eisenberg, Leon (1962) "If Not Now, When?" *American Journal of Orthopsychiatry,* 32:781-793 (October).

Eissler, Kurt (1965) *Medical Orthodoxy and the Future of Psychoanalysis.* New York: International Universities Press.

Ellison, Ralph (1952) *Invisible Man.* New York: Random House.

Engel, George L. (1962) *Psychological Development in Health and Disease.* Philadelphia: W. B. Saunders Company.

Erikson, Erik H. (1950) *Childhood and Society,* ill. rev. ed. New York: W. W. Norton, Inc., 1968.

Felix, Robert H. (1963) "Community Mental Health," *American Journal of Orthopsychiatry,* 33:788-794 (October).

Foucault, Michel (1961) *Madness and Civilization: A History of Insanity in the Age of Reason.* New York: Random House, 1965.

Fox, Robin (1964) "Witchcraft and Clanship in Cochiti Therapy," *Magic, Faith and Healing: Studies in Primitive Psychiatry Today.* Ari Kiev, ed. New York: The Free Press.

Frank, Jerome (1961) *Persuasion and Healing: A Comparative Study of Psychotherapy.* Baltimore: Johns Hopkins Press.

Freedman, Alfred M. (1963) "Beyond Action for Mental Health," *American Journal of Orthopsychiatry,* 33:799-805 (October).

Freud, Sigmund (1893) "Some Points in a Comparative Study of Organic and Hysterical Paralysis," *The Collected Papers of Sigmund Freud,* Vol. I Ernest Jones, ed. London: Hogarth Press, 1956.

———— (1923) *The Ego and the Id.* New York: W. W. Norton and Company, Inc., 1962.

———— (1925) *An Autobiographical Study.* James Strachey transl. New York: W. W. Norton, 1952.

———— (1926) *The Question of Lay Analysis.* James Strachey transl., ed. New York: Doubleday Anchor Books, 1964.

———— (1927) "Postscript to a Discussion on Lay Analysis," *The Collected Papers of Sigmund Freud,* Vol. V. Ernest Jones, ed. pp. 205-214. London: Hogarth Press, 1956.

———— (1930) *Civilization and Its Discontents.* Garden City, New York: Doubleday and Company, Inc., 1958.

Fromm, Erich (1944) "Individual and Social Origins of Neurosis," *American Sociological Review* 9:380-384 (Aug.)

———— (1959) *Sigmund Freud's Mission: An Analysis of His Personality and Influence.* New York: Grove Press.

Glaser, Frederick B. (1965) "The Dichotomy Game: A Further Consideration of the Writings of Dr. Thomas Szasz," *American Journal of Psychiatry,* 121:1069-1074 (May).

Goffman, Erving (1961) *Asylums: Essays on the Social Situation of Mental Patients and Other Inmates.* Garden City, New York: Doubleday and Company, Inc.

Goldston, Stephen E. (1965) "Selected Definitions," *Concepts of Community Psychiatry: A Framework for Training.* Stephen E. Goldston, ed. Public Health Service Publication No. 1319. Bethesda, Maryland: National Institute of Mental Health.

Goodman, Paul (1962) *Growing Up Absurd: Problems of Youth in an Organized Society.* New York: Random House.

Gorman, Mike (1956) *Every Other Bed.* New York: World Publishing Company.

Group for the Advancement of Psychiatry (1954) *Criminal Re-*

sponsibility and Psychiatric Expert Testimony. Report No. 26 New York: Group for the Advancement of Psychiatry.

———— (1962) *The Preclinical Teaching of Psychiatry.* Report No. 54 New York: Group for the Advancement of Psychiatry.

———— (1966) *Psychiatry and Public Affairs.* Chicago: Aldine.

Guttmacher, Manfred S. (1964) "Critique of Views of Thomas Szasz on Legal Psychiatry," *Archives of General Psychiatry,* 10: 239-245 (March).

Haines, William H. and Zeidler John (1958) "Not Guilty by Reason of Insanity," *Crime and Insanity.* Richard W. Nice, ed. New York: Philosophical Library.

Halleck, Seymour (1967) "Psychiatric Management of Dangerous Behavior on a University Campus," *American Journal of Psychiatry,* 124:203-310 (September).

Hart, H. L. A. (1960) "The Ascription of Responsibility and Rights," Anthony Flew, ed. *Logic and Language.* (First Series) Oxford: Basil Blackwell.

———— (1961) *Punishment and the Elimination of Responsibility.* London: Athlone Press.

Hayek, Frederich A. (1944) *The Road to Serfdom.* Chicago: The University of Chicago Press.

Henry, George W. (1941) "Mental Hospitals," Zilboorg, Gregory and Henry, George W. *A History of Medical Psychology.* New York: W. W. Norton and Company, Inc.

Hobbs, Nicholas (1964) "Mental Health's Third Revolution," *American Journal of Orthopsychiatry,* 34:882.

Hollingshead, August B. and Redlich Frederich C. (1958) *Social Class and Mental Illness: A Community Study* New York: John Wiley and Sons.

Holt, Robert (1965) "A Review of Some of Freud's Biological Assumptions and Their Influence on His Theories," *Psychoanalysis and Current Biological Thought.* Norman S. Greenfield and William C. Lewis, eds. Madison, Wisconsin: University of Wisconsin Press, 93-125.

Horowitz, Irving Louis (1967) *The Rise and Fall of Project Camelot: Studies in the Relationship Between Social Science and Practical Politics.* Cambridge, Mass.: The MIT Press.

Hunter, Edward (1956) *Brainwashing.* New York: The Bookmailer.

Jahoda, Marie (1958) *Current Concepts of Positive Mental Health.* New York: Basic Books.

Joint Commission on Mental Illness and Mental Health (1960) *Community Resources in Mental Health.* Monograph Series No. 5 New York: Basic Books.

—— (1961) *Action for Mental Health*. New York: Basic Books.

Jones, Ernest (1953) *The Life and Work of Sigmund Freud: The Formative Years and the Great Discoveries 1856-1900*. Vol. I. New York: Basic Books.

—— (1955) *The Life and Work of Sigmund Freud: Years of Maturity, 1901-1919*, Vol. II, New York: Basic Books.

Jones, Maxwell (1952) *Social Psychiatry: A Study of Therapeutic Communities*. London: Tavistock Publications.

Kahler, Erich (1957) *The Tower and the Abyss: An Inquiry into the Transformation of the Individual*. New York: George Braziller, Inc.

Keniston, Kenneth (1960) "Alienation and the Decline of Utopia," *Varieties of Modern Social Theory*. Hendrik M. Ruitenbeek, ed. New York: E. P. Dutton and Company, Inc., 1963.

Kennedy, John F. (1964) "Message from the President of the United States Relative to Mental Illness and Mental Retardation, February 5, 1963," *American Journal of Psychiatry*, 120:729-737 (February).

Kesey, Ken (1962) *One Flew Over the Cuckoo's Nest*. New York: Viking Press.

Kety, Seymour S. (1965) "Biochemical Theories of Schizophrenia," *International Journal of Psychiatry*, 1:409-430 (July).

King, Lester (1954) "What Is Disease?" *Philosophy of Science* 21:193-203 (July).

Kluckhohn, Clyde (1949) "The Limitations of Adaptation and Adjustment as Concepts for Understanding Cultural Behavior," *Adaptation*. John Romano, ed., Ithaca: Cornell University Press.

Laing, R. D. (1967) *The Politics of Experience*. New York: Pantheon Books.

Langer, Suzanne (1942) *Philosophy in a New Key*. Cambridge: Harvard University Press.

Leifer, Ronald (1963) "The Competence of the Psychiatrist to Assist in the Determination of Incompetency—A Skeptical Inquiry into the Courtroom Functions of Psychiatrists," *Syracuse Law Review*, 14: 564-575 (Summer).

—— (1964a) "Psychiatry, Domestic Tranquility and International Tension," Paper presented to the First International Congress of Social Psychiatry August, 1964, London, England.

—— (1964b) "The Psychiatrist and Tests of Criminal Responsibility," *American Psychologist*, 19:825-830 (November).

—— (1966a) "Psychotherapy, Scientific Method and Ethics," *American Journal of Psychotherapy*. 2:295-304 (April).

—— (1966b) "Community Psychiatry and Social Power," *Social Problems* 14:16-22 (Summer).

———— (1966c) *"Dubious Bridges: Book Review of Psychoanalysis and Current Biological Thought,"* Norman S. Greenfield and William C. Lewis, eds. *Journal of Individual Psychology,* 22:245-247 (November).

———— (1967a) "The Concept of Criminal Responsibility," *ETC: A Review of General Semantics,* 24:177-190 (June).

———— (1967b) "Social Influences on Psychiatric Thought," *The Pharos of Alpha Omega Alpha,* 30:93-96 (July).

———— (1969) "Psychiatry in the Schools," *The Culture of Schools.* Stanley Diamond, ed. New York: Basic Books.

Levine, Alexander (1967) "The Cold War Between Psychiatry and Psychology: A Psychiatrist's View," *Psychiatric Opinion,* 4:5 (June).

Levi-Strauss, Claude (1955) *Tristes-Tropique: An Anthropological Study of Primitive Societies in Brazil.* New York: Atheneum, 1964.

Levitt, Morton (1960) *Freud and Dewey on the Nature of Man.* New York: Philosophical Library.

Lockman, Robert F. (1966) "Nationwide Study Yields Profile of Psychiatrists," *Psychiatric News,* 1:2 (January).

Louch, A. R. (1966) *Explanation and Human Action.* Berkeley: University of California Press.

Lowie, Robert H. (1920) *Primitive Society.* New York: Boni and Liveright.

Maine, Henry Sumner (1861) *Ancient Law: Its Connection with the Early History of Society and Its Relation to Modern Ideas.* Boston: Beacon Press, 1963.

Major Provisions of The New Legislation Governing One Hospitalization of One Mentally Ill. New York State Department of Mental Hygiene, 1965.

Malamud, William and Braceland, Francis J. (1966) "Community Mental Health: Introduction," *American Journal of Psychiatry,* 122:977-978 (March).

Mannheim, Karl (1929) *Ideology and Utopia: An Introduction to the Sociology of Knowledge.* New York: Harcourt, Brace and World, 1936.

Marcuse, Herbert (1955) *Eros and Civilization: A Philosophical Inquiry into Freud.* Boston: Beacon Press.

Mariner, Allen (1967) "A Critical Look at Professional Education in the Mental Health Field," *American Psychologist,* 22:271-281 (April).

McKinney, John C. and Loomis, Charles P. (1957) "The Application of Gemeinschaft and Gesellschaft as Related to Other Typologies:

The Typological Tradition," Tonnie's Ferdinand *Community and Society*. Charles P. Loomis, ed., New York: Harper & Row.

McMillan, John J. (1965) "State and Professional Affairs: Insurance Reimbursement," *American Psychologist* 20:800-801.

———— (1966) "State and Professional Affairs : Psychology and Health Insurance," *American Psychologist* 21:574-575 (June).

M'Naghton's Case (1843) 10 Cl and Fin 200, 8 Eng. Rep 718.

Meachum, Stewart (1964) "The Social Aspects of Nuclear Anxiety," *American Journal of Psychiatry* 120:837-841 (March).

Meadows, Paul (1966) "The Cure of Souls and the Winds of Change," Department of Sociology, Maxwell Graduate School, Syracuse University (Mimeographed).

Menninger, Karl (1961) *The Theory of Psychoanalytic Technique*. New York: Science Editions.

Mental Illness and Due Process (1962) Report and Recommendations on Admission to Mental Hospitals Under New York Law by the Special Committee to Study Committment Procedures of the Association of the Bar of New York City. Ithaca: Cornell University Press.

The Mentally Disabled and the Law: Report of the American Bar Foundation on the Rights of the Mentally Ill (1961). Lindman, Frank T. and McIntyre, Donald M. eds., Chicago: University of Chicago Press.

Mills, C. Wright (1940) "Situated Actions and Vocabularies of Motive," *American Sociological Review* 46:316-330 (November).

Miner, Horace (1956) "Body Ritual Among the Nacirema," *American Anthropologist* 58:503-507.

Morris, Charles W. (1938) "Foundations of the Theory of Signs," *International Encyclopedia of Unified Science*. Vol. I., Otto Neurath, Rudolph Carnap and Charles Morris, Chicago: The University of Chicago Press, 77-137.

Morris, Charles W. (1946) *Signs, Language and Behavior*. New Jersey: Prentice-Hall.

Muller, Herbert J. (1961) *Freedom in the Ancient World*. New York: Harper & Row.

Myers, Jerome K. and Roberts, Bertram H. (1959) *Family and Class Dynamics in Mental Illness*. New York: John Wiley.

Nelson, Benjamin (1965). "Self Image and Systems of Spiritual Direction in the History of European Civilization," *The Quest for Self-Control: Classical Philosophies and Scientific Research*. S. Z. Kalusner, ed., New York: The Free Press.

Neumann, Erich (1954) *The Origins and History of Consciousness*. Bollingen Foundation Series XLII. New York: Pantheon Books.

Nice, Richard W. ed. (1958) *Crime and Insanity*. New York: Philosophical Library.

Nietzsche, Friedrich (1885) *Thus Spake Zarathustra*. New York: The Modern Library.

Nisbet, Robert (1962) *Community and Power*. New York: Oxford University Press.

Noyes, Arthur P. and Kolb, Lawrence C. (1958) *Modern Clinical Psychiatry*. Philadelphia: W. B. Saunders.

"Number of Mental Hospital Patients Drops 11th Straight Year, PHS Notes" (1967) *Medical Tribune*, Vol. 8 No. 86, August 17, p. 4.

Oberndorf, C. P. (1953) *A History of Psychoanalysis in America*. New York: Grune and Stratton.

Offer, Daniel and Sabshin, Melvin (1966) *Normality: Theoretical and Clinical Concepts of Mental Health*. New York: Basic Books.

Ozarin, Lucy D. and Brown, Bertram S. (1965) "New Directions and Community Mental Health Programs," *American Journal of Orthopsychiatry*, 35:10-17 (January).

Parsons, Talcott (1951a) *The Social System*. Glencoe, Illinois: The Free Press of Glencoe.

―――― (1951b) "Illness and the Role of the Physician: A Sociological Perspective," *American Journal of Orthopsychiatry*, 21:452-560 (July).

―――― (1958b) "Social Structure and the Development of Personality: Freud's Contribution to the Integration of Psychology and Sociology," *Psychiatry*, 21:321-340 (November).

―――― (1958b) "Definitions of Health and Illness in the Light of American Values and Social Structure," *Social Structure and Personality*. New York: The Free Press, 1964.

Perlin, Seymour and Kahn Robert L. (1963) "The Overlap of Medical and Non-Medical Institutions in Community Mental Health Programs," *Comprehensive Psychiatry*, 4:461-467 (December).

Peters, R. S., (1958) *The Concept of Motivation*. London: Routledge and Kegan Paul.

Pinel, Philippe (1806) *A Treatise on Insanity*. New York: Hafner Publishing Company, 1962.

Pleune, Gordon (1965) "All Dis-ease Is Not Disease: A Consideration of Psychoanalysis, Psychotherapy and Psycho-social Engineering," *International Journal of Psychoanalysis*, 46:358-366.

Popper, Karl (1934) *The Logic of Scientific Discovery*. London: Hutchinson, 1959.

Presthus, Robert (1962) *The Organization Society: An Analysis and a Theory.* New York: Knopf.

Radin, Paul (1927) *Primitive Man as Philosopher.* 2d rev. ed. New York: D. Appleton and Company, 1967.

—— (1937) *Primitive Religion: Its Nature and Origins.* New York: Dover Publications, Inc., 1957.

Rafferty, Frank T. (1963) "Symptoms and Process in the Multidisciplined Community," *American Journal of Orthopsychiatry,* 33:316 (March).

Rapoport, Anatole (1953) *Operational Philosophy.* New York: Harper and Brothers.

Rapoport, Robert N. (1960) *Community As Doctor: New Perspectives on a Therapeutic Community.* London: Tavistock Publications.

Raskin, M. G. (1964) "Political Anxiety and Nuclear Reality," *American Journal of Psychiatry,* Vol. 120 (March) 120:831-836.

Redfield, Robert (1953) *The Primitive World and Its Transformations.* Ithaca, New York: Cornell University Press.

—— (1956) *The Little Community and Peasant Society and Culture.* Chicago: The University of Chicago Press.

Reichenbach, Hans (1947) *Elements of Symbolic Logic.* New York: MacMillan.

Research Conference on Therapeutic Community (1960) Herman C. B. Denber ed., Springfield, Illinois: Charles C. Thomas.

Riessman, Frank and Hallowitz, Emanuel (1967) "The Neighborhood Service Center: An Innovation in Prevention Psychiatry," *American Journal of Psychiatry* 123:1408-1413 (May).

Riessman, Frank and Scribner, Sylvia (1965) "The Under-Utilization of Mental Health Services by Workers and Low Income Groups: Causes and Cures," *American Journal of Psychiatry,* 121:789-801.

Robinson, David (1966). *Summary of Pertinent Aspects of Community Mental Health Centers Legislation.* (Mimeographed)

Rosen, George (1956) "Hospitals, Medical Care and Social Policy in the French Revolution," *Bulletin of the History of Medicine,* 30:124-149 (March-April).

—— (1959) "Social Stress and Mental Disease from the Eighteenth Century to the Present: Some Origins of Social Psychiatry," *Milbank Memorial Fund Quarterly* 37:5-32 (January).

—— (1963) "Social Attitudes to Irrationality and Madness in 17th and 18th Century Europe," *Journal of the History of Medicine and Allied Sciences,* 18:220-240 (July).

—— (1964) "The Mentally Ill and the Community in Western and Central Europe During the Late Middle Ages and the

Renaissance," *Journal of the History of Medicine* 19:377-388 (October).

Ryle, Gilbert (1949) *The Concept of Mind.* New York: Barnes and Noble.

Sachar, Edward (1966). "Criminal Law and Behavioral Science," Slovenko, Ralph, ed. *Crime, Law and Corrections* Springfield, Illinois: Charles C. Dranos.

Sachlins, Marshall (1967) "The Established Order: Do Not Fold, Spindle or Mutilate," *The Rise and Fall of Project Camelot,* Irving Louis Horowitz, ed. Cambridge: MIT Press.

Sandt, John J. and Leifer, Ronald (1964) "The Psychiatric Consultation," *Comprehensive Psychiatry,* 5:409-418 (December).

Schein, Edgar H. (1961) *Coercive Persuasion.* New York: W. W. Norton.

Schiller, F. C. S. (1903) "The Ethical Basis of Metaphysics," *Humanism, Philosophical Essays.* 2d ed. rev. London: Macmillan, 1921.

Schur, Edwin M. (1966) "Psychiatrists Under Attack: The Rebellious Dr. Szasz," *Atlantic Monthly.*

Seeman, Melvin (1959) "On the Meaning of Alienation," *American Sociological Review,* 24:783-790 (December).

Shoben, Edward Joseph (1953) "Some Observations on Psychotherapy and the Learning Process." *Psychotherapy: Theory and Research* O. Hobert Mowrer, ed. New York: The Ronald Press.

Sigerist, Henry E. (1960) *On the History of Medicine.* Felix Marti Ibancz, ed. New York: M.D. Publications.

Smith, M. Brewster and Hobbs, Nicholas (1966) "The Community and the Community Mental Health Center," *American Psychologist* 21:499-509 (June).

Sulzer, Edward (1962) "Reinforcement and the Therapeutic Contract." *Journal of Counselling Psychology* 9:271-276 (Fall).

Szasz, Thomas S. (1956) "Malingering: 'Diagnosis' or Social Condemnation?" *AMA Archives of Neurology and Psychiatry,* 76:432-443 (October).

———— (1957a) *Pain and Pleasure.* New York: Basic Books.

———— (1957b) "Some Observations on the Use of Tranquilizing Drugs," *AMA Archives of Neurology and Psychiatry,* 77:96-108 (January).

———— (1957c) "Commitment of the Mentally Ill 'Treatment' or Social Restraint?" *Journal of Nervous and Mental Disease,* 125:293-307 (April-June).

———— (1957d) "On the Theory of Psychoanalytic Treatment," *International Journal of Psychoanalysis* 38:166-182.

———— (1958) "Politics and Mental Health: Some Remarks Apropos of the Case of Mr. Ezra Pound," *American Journal of Psychiatry*, 115:508-511 (December).

———— (1960) "Civil Liberties and Mental Illness Some Observations on the Case of Miss Edith L. Hough," *Journal of Nervous and Mental Disease*, 131:58-63 (July).

———— (1961a) *The Myth of Mental Illness: Foundations of a Theory of Personal Conduct*. New York: Hoeber-Harper.

———— (1961b) "The Uses of Naming and the Origin of the Myth of Mental Illness," *American Psychologist* 16:59-65 (February).

———— (1961c) "Criminal Responsibility and Psychiatry," Hans Toch (ed.) *Legal and Criminal Psychology* New York: Holt, Rinehart and Winston, Inc.

———— (1961b) "Hospital-Patient Relationships in Medicine and Psychiatry," *Mental Hygiene*, 45:171-179 (April).

———— (1963) *Law, Liberty and Psychiatry*. New York: MacMillan.

———— (1964) "Psychoanalysis and Taxation," *American Journal of Psychotherapy*, 18:635-643 (October).

———— (1965a) *Psychiatric Justice*. New York: MacMillan.

———— (1965b) *The Ethics of Psychoanalysis: The Theory and Method of Autonomous Psychotherapy*. New York: Basic Books, Inc.

———— (1966a) "The Mental Health Ethic," *Ethics and Society: Original Essays on Contemporary Moral Problems*. Richard T. DeGeorge ed. Garden City, New York: Doubleday Anchor Books.

———— (1966b) "Psychotherapy: A Sociocultural Perspective," *Comprehensive Psychiatry*, 7:217:223 (August).

Tarsis, Valery (1965) *Ward Seven: An Autobiographical Novel* Katya Brown, transl. 1st ed. New York: Dutton.

Thompkins, Harvey J. (1967) "The Presidential Address: The Physician in Contemporary Society," *American Journal of Psychiatry*, 124:1-6 (July).

Thorne, Frederick C. (1966) "An Analysis of Szasz' 'Myth of Mental Illness,'" *American Journal of Psychiatry* 123:652-656 (December).

Tillich, Paul (1961) "The Meaning of Health," *Perspectives in Biology and Medicine*, 5:92-100 (Autumn).

Tonnies, Ferdinand (1887) *Community and Society*. Charles P. Loomis, transl and ed. East Lansing: Michigan State University Press, 1957.

Tocqueville, Alex (1836) *Democracy in America*. Henry Reeve, transl. rev. ed. New York: Oxford University Press, 1947.

Turbayne, Colin M. (1962) *The Myth of Metaphor*. New Haven: Yale University Press.

Visotsky, Harold (1964) "Social Psychiatry Rationale: Administrative and Planning Approaches," *American Journal of Psychiatry*, 121: 433-441 (December).
—— (1965) "Community Psychiatry: We Are Willing to Learn," *American Journal of Psychiatry* 122:696-693 (December).

Vahanian, Gabriel (1957) *The Death of God: The Culture of Our Post Christian Era.* New York: George Braziller.

Weihofen, Henry (1954) *Mental Disorder as a Criminal Defense* Buffalo: Dennis and Company.

Weiss, Paul (1949) "The Biological Basis of Adaptation," *Adaptation.* John Romano, ed. Ithaca: Cornell University Press.

Wheelis, Allen (1958) *The Quest for Identity.* New York: W. W. Norton, Inc.

White, Leslie A. (1959) *The Evolution of Culture: The Development of Civilization to the Fall of Rome.* New York: McGraw Hill Book Company, Inc.

Whitehorn, John C. (1963) "The Doctor's Image of Man," *Man's Image in Medicine and Anthropology.* Iago Goldston, ed. New York: International Universities Press.

Wittgenstein, Ludwig (1953) *Philosophical Investigations.* G.E.M. Anscombe transl. 2d ed. New York: MacMillan.

Woodger, J. H. (1956) *Physics, Psychology and Medicine: A Methodological Essay.* Cambridge: Cambridge University Press.

Zilboorg, Gregory and Henry, George W. (1941) *A History of Medical Psychology.* New York: W. W. Norton & Co.

Zwerling, Israel (1965) *Some Implications of Social Psychiatry for Psychiatric Treatment and Patient Care.* Strecker Monograph Series No. 2, Philadelphia: The Institute of Pennsylvania Hospital.

Index